CHANGE AND TEAMWORK IN PRIMARY CARE

CHANGE AND TEAMWORK IN PRIMARY CARE

Edited by
MIKE PRINGLE, FRCGP
Senior Lecturer, Department of General Practice
University of Nottingham

Published by the BMJ Publishing Group
Tavistock Square, London WC1H 9JR

First published 1993

British Library Cataloguing in Publication Data

Change and Teamwork in Primary Care.

I. Pringle, Mike
362. 172068

ISBN 0–7279–0779–4

The following picture sources are acknowledged:

Hulton Picture Company, page 59; Susan Wilson, pages 66, 114; Sally and Richard Greenhill, pages 72, 82; J Twinning, page 87; John Rae, page 87; Sue de Jong/Format, page 105.

Typeset by Bedford Typesetters Limited, Bedford
Printed and bound in Great Britain by
Latimer Trend & Company Ltd, Plymouth

Contents

Partners in Practice

Introduction

When the NHS was created in 1948 primary care was seen as a necessary appendage to the real site of medical care—the hospitals—and its main role was seen to be that of a triage system to filter out self limiting and minor illness. Until the general practice charter in 1966 primary care was in the doldrums, deprived of resources and respect. The charter created many features of general practice today, including the partial reimbursement of rents, rates, and staffing, and incentives for group practices. For many doctors this was a time of considerable change, but one they largely welcomed. The changes were, by and large, seen to be for the better.

The next 20 years saw a remarkable evolution within primary care. The ugly duckling metamorphosed into a triumph of socialised medicine—quality care accessible to everybody. This period had its fair share of change, of course, including the introduction of items of service payments, vocational training, the teaching of medical students, and the formation of primary health care teams. It was, however, an era in which practices developed opportunistically in response to the incentives and culture of an evolving health service.

Without doubt we are now in turbulent times. Although the government's consultative document on primary care in 1986 clearly acknowledged the extraordinary development in primary care over two decades, it ushered in a period of imposed change from which we are all still reeling. Neighbourhood nursing came first as a stalking horse for the new contract. These were followed by *Working for Patients*, *Caring for People*, and the *Health of the Nation*.

There were parts of this avalanche of imposed changes that were widely welcomed. Medical audit was thought to be the medical equivalent to motherhood and apple pie, while the setting of public health objectives in the *Health of the Nation* was felt both appropriate and overdue. As their full implications for primary care become evident, even these may be seen as two edged swords.

As the Department of Health lurched from indirect to direct management of primary care, the demands made on general practitioners, nurses, and employed staff increased dramatically—and morale plummeted. But in the mid-1980s there was a common perception that "something must be done." General practice was splitting into two camps, with one offering a substandard service. Hospitals were seen as uncontrolled and uncontrollable. Extra resources seemed only to fuel waiting lists and increase stories of poor patient service.

It is not my task in this introduction to reflect on the wisdom of the changes imposed, or to comment on their success or otherwise. It is important, however, to see recent events, as this book does, in two dimensions. The first is the dimension of change itself.

Although the recent upheavals have been extreme, all practices have always been encountering change. Some has been internally generated by, for example, the need to change the appointments system or appoint a new receptionist. Some is imposed locally by, for example, the decision of a partner to retire. Much has always been externally imposed through changes to the Statement of Fees and Allowances.

There have always been individual doctors and practices with special skills in managing these changes, and they had a competitive edge over those that floundered. The difference at the end of the day did not seem especially great since general practice has always made an art form of "muddling by." In the past five years the practices with the skills to manage change have had a pronounced advantage. They were early users of computers and had good information systems; they valued practice management and had high quality practice managers; they understood resources and planning and were able to become fundholders.

General practice is now at the centre of the health service. This has been shown by the special status and power that contracting has bestowed, and by the extra resources that are coming our way. It was dramatically shown by the Tomlinson report, which has recommended that London hospitals be closed and the money transferred to primary care, an idea unthinkable 10 years ago. But this emphasis on primary care puts special responsibilities and pressures on practices. Those unable to respond will be marginalised while the others will be rewarded. This is not to justify or applaud the changes, but only to reflect the reality of today. Those practices with skills in the management of change will be winners—that is abundantly clear. The first half of this book describes some of those skills and how to apply them.

The second dimension to the current changes involves a shift in our working patterns. To maximise income from the new contract most practices have introduced health promotion clinics, visits to elderly people, new registration medicals, and minor surgery—all done or assisted by practice nurses. The new demands on practice information systems in annual reports, business plans, and resource bids have increased the need for adminstrative support, and fundholding has exposed many weakness in practice management.

From April 1993 community nursing staff are included in fundholding budgets and soon the term "attached staff" will disappear from our vocabulary. We are on the threshold of the creation of the primary health care teams that we dreamed of through the 1970s and 1980s. These new teams will require new skills in organisation and communication as part of the evolving culture of practices. Then there will be a need to redefine roles and responsibilities. The days of the medical hegemony are numbered. General practitioners will no longer be the ruling class of primary care. Even the term "partnership" will need to evolve to encompass a more democratic and egalitarian working relationship throughout the primary health care team.

This, then, is the subject of the second part of this book. A number of experts from primary care examine the tasks and relationships that will mould this new partnership. These dual challenges—to control change and adapt our working relationships—are pivotal in primary care today. The manner in which practices react to and master these challenges will determine the success or failure of the new health service. And to that extent it will determine whether the very existence of a public health service continues to be a viable political option.

M PRINGLE

Managing Change
in
Primary Care

Managing change in general practice

MIKE PRINGLE

There is a popular myth, especially evident among politicians, that general practice is ultraconservative. Little has changed over the years and little will change in the foreseeable future. We are, in short, a cold bed of Luddites.

This misconception derives, I believe, from the fact that, as in all professions, new ideas are treated with healthy scepticism until their worth is evident. Once adopted by a large minority, however, innovations quickly become the norm. Politicians are uncomfortable with this. If they encourage changes they are usually experimented with, evaluated, and, finally, after some time, may be adopted. This makes change unpredictable and slow, so they often opt for a second course, imposition, which in its turn creates problems of acceptance and morale.

The reality is, as every practitioner knows, that change is endemic in general practice—it just may not happen in the way that outsiders would wish. On reflecting back over the past 10 years in our practice the evidence is stark. We have moved from an extension on the back of the then senior partner's house to a purpose built medical centre. Staffing has increased from just two dispensers to include a manager, secretary, data analyst, two practice nurses, and a cohort of receptionists and dispensers. We have seen the arrival of an internal telephone system, pagers, computers, nebulisers, electrocardiographs, defibrillators, and sonic aids. The clinical work has changed from being almost totally reactive to planned care for chronic disease and a pervasive emphasis on prevention. We now have vocational

3

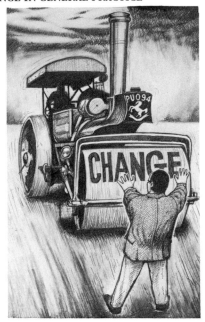

trainees and students; a patient participation group and annual reports; medical audit; and prescribing formularies.

These changes have been replicated throughout general practice, but their evolutionary nature precludes the announcement of a revolution. We need to sensitise ourselves to the degree of change that we have been involved in, and to proclaim it to the world outside.

How well do general practitioners manage change?

To many practices change is something that happens to them. It is an uncontrollable steam roller that thunders over them, always leaving destruction in its wake. This sense of passivity was clearly illustrated to me during a weekend meeting in March 1990, just a month before the new contract was imposed. There were a number of general practitioners and practice managers who had done no preparation. They had not begun to organise their preventive care to achieve the targets, or to plan for visits to elderly people. They were staring at the front wheel of the steam roller, mesmerised.

There are, however, other practices that view change as a challenge which will yield opportunities—in even the most desperate of circumstances something can be gained. These practices set out to manage the change that confronts them, not necessarily with total success, as this example illustrates.

Example 1

When our long serving practice manager announced her intention of retiring, the partners had a series of meetings at which we decided to extend the management skills in the practice and to appoint someone with experience in industry. A job description was drawn up, which included many management tasks which were either new to us or traditionally the responsibility of the partners. An improved pay and holiday package was devised and agreed (on the basis of the new job definition) with the family health services authority.

A personnel officer from a major bank was recruited to teach us shortlisting and interviewing skills. In the interviews each partner had a set of predetermined and standardised questions designed to explore attitudes, skills, and knowledge. The result was substantially more satisfying and successful than any previous appointment process, and an excellent candidate was appointed.

We then discovered that our outgoing practice manager was feeling hurt and betrayed. Not only had we seemed to relish the task of appointing her successor, betraying no evidence of her indispensability, but we were offering better pay and conditions. She felt that all her years of service were being undervalued.

Discussion Virtually any problem can be turned into an opportunity. By thinking about the process of change, the change can be managed so that the chances of a good result are increased. The partnership shared common objectives and acknowledged, and rectified, deficiencies in its skills. We let ourselves down, however, in communication skills and understanding. The outgoing practice manager should have been encouraged to share in the upgrading of her post, preferably by being made to feel that it was her idea, and the partners should have been more sensitive to her self esteem.

Can general practitioners learn how to manage change?

A medical degree appears to confer on a person a God given ability to manage. Within a few years the doctor is a partner in a practice with a turnover of hundreds of thousands of pounds, or perhaps a consultant in an independent hospital trust responsible for a substantial budget. While it is often accepted that skills in personnel, budgeting and finance, and project management are necessary and can be acquired, they are seldom taught. The management of change is usually totally ignored.

Many changes, especially in the past few years, are imposed from outside the practice or by unavoidable circumstances within it—such as the retirement of the manager—and the task is to minimise the disruption while maximising the benefit. Equally, many changes come voluntarily from within the practice—for example, computerisation, upgrading of premises, and vocational training. The task remains the same but the circumstances differ. The partners and practice manager are often now "imposing" the change on the practice and need to be sensitive to issues of presentation, timing, and communication.

Industry and commerce have been aware of this for many years. There are lots of lessons that are transferable to medicine, and particularly to primary care. Some of these skills, or their absence, are illustrated in this second example.

Example 2

Our computer system needed replacing. The new system was delivered and the partners envisaged a steady changeover, with the two computers running in parallel for some time. The system offered the facility, new to us, of prescribing in the consultation, so the partners began to use it with considerable enthusiasm.

The dispensary staff were told about the new computer but were not involved in its choice. They had minimal training, but initially all went smoothly. They found using one system for repeat and one for acute prescribing difficult, but they coped remarkably well. As the repeat prescriptions were transferred to the new system they had added difficulties through the transition but still did not complain.

It then became apparent that the new system's prescription queue for dispensing did not function correctly. Patients were ordering drugs, which were entered on the queue, but if they went too near the bottom that was where they stayed. When the patients came for their drugs they had not been dispensed. Our dispensers took all the flak for a teething problem in a computer system they had not chosen and towards which they felt no loyalty. The resulting crisis required considerable time before solutions were found and the staff felt happier with the new system.

Discussion   The partners owned the new computer both financially and emotionally. This was not important so long as the introduction

---

Points to note

- Change is endemic in general practice
- The need for change can be turned into an opportunity
- Change may be imposed from outside or come from within the practice
- Appropriate management of change increases the chance of a good result
- All members of a practice should be involved in the management of change
- The appointment of a practice manager should reduce the partners' responsibility for managing change

---

was relatively smooth, but once problems occurred the lack of staff commitment to the project was exposed. Goodwill alone is not sufficient, people need to feel an emotional investment in the success of an innovation. If the staff had taken a greater part in making the decisions on the choice of computer and its introduction then the trauma and the extra hours resolving the crisis would have been avoided.

Who should do the managing?

There is an evident transition occurring between administration and management in general practice. The old model of internal promotion of a senior receptionist to take on administrative responsibility with the misnomer of "practice manager" is giving way to the appointment of people, often from outside the health service, with management skills. This was illustrated in the first example given above.

This is not to say that partners will or should surrender their responsibilities for the future of their practices. The evolving model is one in which the partners and practice manager decide broad strategy (for example, whether premises should be extended) but the practice manager supervises the process, reporting back to the practice meeting on progress. This delegation requires skills of a high order from the partners if it is not to become an abdication.

And the new practice managers, who may be receiving profit related pay, will require high level skills to fulfil the expectations of

7

the partners and the practice. As our contract, our task, and our bureaucratic relationships become more complex so does the job description of the practice manager, but the basic skills for the successful management of change will remain the same.

Conclusion

Change cannot be avoided but it can be managed. This does not mean it becomes painless, but the pain can be mitigated while the benefits are maximised. All members of a practice need to be involved in this management of change, although the appointment of real practice managers should reduce the direct responsibility of the medical partners.

Learning from the past

JUSTIN ALLEN, ANDREW WILSON

Doctors in a three partner practice do all their own on call out of hours work in an equal rota of nights and weekends. The senior partner is aged 56. He has given vague hints that he is planning to retire at 60 but has never confirmed this. His two junior partners have been in the practice for three and four years respectively. At a partners' meeting he announces that he is proposing to give up his night work as he is finding this increasingly irksome, and has done it uninterrupted for the previous 27 years. He is proposing that the change should take effect from the beginning of the next quarter, in six weeks' time. His proposal is that the junior partners would take over his responsibility and in return would share all the income received for night visits. Much to his surprise he is met with an angry refusal. Hurt and rejected by this response, he gets angry and threatens to dissolve the partnership and the meeting breaks up in uproar.

Most practices will be able to recall similar examples of proposed change going wrong. But most can also point to changes that have been successfully implemented and found to be beneficial. Change, or the possibility of it, is with us all the time. This ranges from the major externally imposed upheavals that have been a feature of general practice over the past few years to minor adjustments within the practice. All practices, therefore, have a wealth of experience of change. Can they use these experiences to improve their management of change? According to Socrates, experience has taught our best flautists, but it has also taught our worst. The following questions allow a practice to review its changes over recent years.

9

How much have we changed?

Has the practice been either too stagnant or too unstable? The degree of change and its frequency should be considered. One major change, such as the breaking up of a partnership, might have prolonged repercussions. However, frequent small changes may also have an impact. In industrial settings frequent environmental changes have been shown to boost productivity (the Hawthorne effect). In contrast, general practitioners often complain about the frequency of minor changes, such as to standard referral forms or protocols for child health surveillance.

Have changes been in response to external events or have they been initiated internally? Changes resulting from a perceived need are clearly more likely to be welcomed and are less traumatic and frustrating than those imposed from outside. This also applies within an organisation; although some members of a practice might feel in control of internally generated change, this does not necessarily apply to others.

What is our attitude to change?

It is unlikely that all members of the practice feel the same about the benefit or otherwise of change. In any group some will be good at having new ideas, others at analysing positive and negative features of proposals for change, and others at actually initiating change and making it work. As well as there being such a range of skills, attitudes to change will also differ. Some may be naturally conservative and difficult to persuade that any change is better than the status quo.

- Much can be learnt from practices' experience both of proposed change going wrong and of successful change
- Changes resulting from a perceived need internally are more likely to be welcomed than those imposed from outside
- Practice members will have a wide range of different skills to offer and different attitudes towards change
- There must be a workable structure for decision making and style of management
- The way a change is implemented is important to its success
- The effect of change should be evaluated

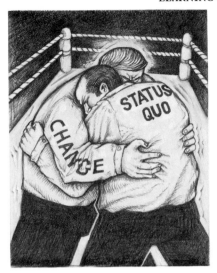

Others may resist change for more pragmatic reasons and argue that it is not worth the disruption it would cause. At the other end of the spectrum some may enjoy the process of change and respond to problems by suggesting a change to the system rather than by trying to make existing arrangements work.

Such a mixture is beneficial to an organisation—if everyone excelled at new ideas but not at following them through little change would occur and all would be frustrated. The benefit of such a mix of skills and attitudes, however, can be realised only if individuals are aware of their own attributes and those of others. Practices may wish to explore this in a formal way by using recognised psychological tests or informally through discussion. As well as differences in attitude, the reaction to change at both individual and practice level will be determined by previous events and current morale. An unsuccessful attempt at change or low morale might leave members feeling bruised and defensive.

How are changes initiated?

However good the mix of talents, change can be successful only if a suitable structure for decision making and management exists. If the past has been too turbulent a practice might conclude that this is because change is initiated too readily, without proper consultation. Alternatively, a practice might decide that too much consultation and attempt to consensus have occurred, resulting in any innovation being squashed. Each practice needs to establish its own style of management and to find a method that suits participants. However, the style has to be agreed; problems will arise if some members think the chosen style is democratic and consultative, while others are working to a more hierarchical system.

As well as style of management, practices should consider whether decisions about change are made at the appropriate level of organisation. Should a practice manager have the sole responsibility to select reception staff? Should a partner's proposal to change the hours of a surgery be discussed with receptionists only after a decision has been reached? Problems may arise if decisions are made at an inappropriate level, or more commonly because no policy has been established on the mechanism to be used.

How has change been implemented?

The implementation of change raises similar issues. Some members of the practice are likely to be better than others at implementing an agreed proposal. The way a change is implemented is a major determinant of its success. How are those not involved in the initial decision informed of the proposal? How much modification is acceptable? How are the fears of those against the proposal dealt with? Changes implemented gradually are less likely to be disruptive but more likely to be frustrating to those in support. Should there be a pilot or trial period? Some new initiatives are bound to fail. What safeguards have been constructed so that if this should happen chaos does not result? It may be worth demonstrating the feasibility of a new system before irrevocably abandoning the old.

How has change been evaluated?

The most neglected aspect of change, particularly by those who enjoy the process, is the assessment of whether the change has been successful. If changes found to be counterproductive are not withdrawn the organisation will rightly become resistant to future initiatives. Evaluation is possible only if there has been a clear statement of the purpose and content of a proposed change. The ultimate objective of a change may be immeasurable—for example, a practice would not be able to show the effect of its new diabetic clinic on mortality and morbidity. However, process and intermediate outcomes are measurable—for example, it would be possible to audit who was invited to the clinic, who attended, and whether designated procedures were followed during the attendance. It is important to consider unpredicted effects of change, and those produced elsewhere in the organisation—the new diabetic clinic may have been very successful in achieving its objectives, but due to overrunning led to unacceptable waiting times in the surgery session which followed it.

What experiences of change can we learn from?

The scenario at the beginning of this chapter is an example of how a proposed change failed. Failure may also arise at a later stage. As well as reviewing change in general, as suggested above, specific attempts at change, successful or unsuccessful, may give further insights into how the practice can work best.

The first consideration is the background to the change—what was the morale of the practice and individuals? Were individuals defensive or confident? Who introduced the proposal, and why, and with what prior consultation? How was the idea introduced, how was it negotiated, and who was consulted? How was a decision about the proposal made and was it unanimous? How was the change implemented and evaluated?

Examples

Below we describe how this process might work, starting with the scenario at the beginning of this chapter. We can perhaps see why this proposal went wrong. Examining the process in detail, in the light of the factors mentioned above, may provide further insights that could help this practice in the future.

Past experience Looking back to the recent past would show that change in the working arrangements in this practice had always proved difficult. Many other proposed changes had been blocked by the senior partner, whose attitude to change had always seemed to favour the status quo. The partners, who were being expected to cover the extra nights on call, had not perceived a need for this change and therefore were unlikely to be keen on it, particularly in the light of their previous experiences. The overall impact of the proposal, the advantages and the drawbacks, had not been considered or discussed, and none of the parties had looked at the issues from their colleagues' point of view. In an attempt to rush things through, the normal decision making rules had been bypassed and actual implementation of the change proposed with immediate and apparently permanent effect.

Introduction of the idea   What might have happened if the factors outlined previously had been taken into account by the partnership concerned? It is, of course, not possible for them to change their recent past. The abruptness of the proposal, however, might have been better handled if the senior partner had introduced the idea at a previous meeting, suggesting its discussion next time. This would allow them all time to get used to the idea of the change. If, in addition, he had given the reasons for the request—he was having problems coping with night calls, particularly since a recent illness— then his partners could start to consider things from his point of view. At the definitive meeting the impact of the proposal could then have been evaluated from all points of view. If any of the parties still had doubts a trial period could be proposed, followed by an evaluation and possible renegotiation. This would allow them all to be reassured that in agreeing to the change they would not prejudice their current position too much. In the event, the partners concerned finally agreed to a plan very similar to this, but only after a further meeting to resolve all the ill feeling previously generated. This partnership decided that in future, when making a major change, they should look at their previous experiences and by planning things better they would not make the same mistakes again.

Improved methods   Moving along a few years we can see the same partnership approaching another major change differently. On this occasion the proposal was to reduce the number of partners in order to improve earning potential. This was made possible by the withdrawal of an existing partner. Early in the deliberations one of the remaining partners suggested that the partnership should consider the advantages of not appointing a replacement. The practice had adopted some quite radical changes in the previous year or so and had coped with them without difficulty. A clear evaluation of the pros and cons was prepared for the partnership meeting, with an analysis of the likely increase in income and a management plan indicating how the extra work was to be dealt with, and this was discussed fully. The impact on individual members of the practice, as well as the whole group, was also considered. An immediate decision was not demanded, and the decision was taken over two or three meetings. A trial period of six months with a full evaluation was proposed from the outset, and the upshot was that the change was implemented without a hitch. Interestingly, the partnership concerned, on reviewing that decision at the end of the trial period, changed its mind and agreed the need for a replacement partner, again without a problem.

Conclusion

In all organisations change is occurring all the time. It may go smoothly, but it may cause problems. If it goes badly wrong it can cause a great deal of stress, often needlessly. By looking back at the way changes have occurred in the past it is possible to identify where things have gone wrong. If lessons can be learnt and then applied the process will be much smoother.

Strategies for success

CHRIS ATKINSON, JACKY HAYDEN

Change in general practice when handled well can be stimulating and rewarding. Improving the practice to benefit patient care and providing care more economically are good for practice morale, which in turn boosts patient care. If change is handled badly, however, it can create anger and resentment and have a negative effect on patient care.

We all like to think that we are doing a good job and most of us would resist criticism; this is particularly true in general practice, which inevitably has considerable personal involvement and investment. Introducing change in general practice can often be met with considerable resistance.

A problem may become obvious in a practice in various different ways: a crisis may occur, such as a preventable death, which may highlight a deficiency in practice organisation; one or more partners may have experienced a new way of working; or the practice as a whole may decide that external forces, such as the new general practitioner contract and alteration in patient demography, have created a need for change. Alternatively, the practice might undertake systematic audit and identify deficiencies in its systems, holding regular management meetings to identify and implement change.

Vision sharing

Working in a general practice is like working in any other team—if all members of the health care team are involved in determining the character of the practice they are more likely to be committed to those

16

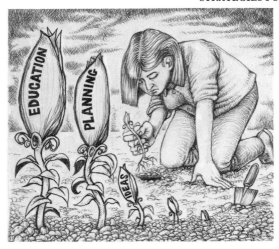

ideals and to implement them.[1] Alternatively, introducing change without consultation may result in members of the team obstructing the proposed change. Consultation must, however, ensure that all members of the practice understand the new process, as shown by the following example.

Example 1

A practice decided to introduce dietetic services for the local population. The doctors and practice manager met with the dietitian and planned the introduction of the service; reception staff were consulted and were in agreement. The service was popular with the patients but conflict arose within the practice because one member of the reception staff had failed to understand that the service was for all the local population, not just the patients registered with the practice. She resented local inhabitants other than those registered with the practice using the service, apparently taking care away from the practice population.

Strategy meetings

The first stage in managing change is to define the overall aim of the practice. It is important that everyone involved in the practice is able to share in this stage. In a small practice it may be possible for all the practice team to work in a single group, each having an opportunity to express his or her views on their ideal practice. In a large practice this process may need to involve only a limited number of the team—

17

perhaps the doctors, practice nurse, and practice manager—as when a meeting is too large individuals are inhibited from contributing. An important preliminary step, however, is for this group to listen to all the other team members and to share the results of the smaller meeting with everyone concerned.

Such strategic thinking will need time. One way of ensuring that the meeting is uninterrupted is to hold it away from the practice, perhaps for a whole day.

Where is practice now and where does it want to be?

When the broad aims of the practice have been identified the team needs to think through the individual components and set out a series of objectives which are manageable. At this stage it is advisable to identify one or two people who will have responsibility for a specific area. Identifying a date for reporting back will prevent procrastination.

As general practice is such a vast topic it may be helpful to think in

---

Cervical cytology uptake

Where are we now?
50% Uptake, poor information about women who have had a hysterectomy

Factors maintaining status quo
Apathy
Patient rights
Lack of knowledge
Inadequate equipment
Lack of time

What do we need to change?
1 Identification of risk group
2 Increased availability of cervical cytology
3 Attitude of doctors to taking smears

Where do we want to be?
80% Or greater uptake in women in whom cervical cytology is indicated

Factors facilitating change
Financial gain
Good practice
Peer pressure
Patient pressure

---

the areas defined by the Royal College of General Practitioners: professional values, availability and accessibility, clinical competence, and communication.[2] This framework should prevent large areas being ignored or forgotten. Each of the four areas will need considerable expansion, and it may be that only one can be managed at a time.

Each problem can be considered in detail. The group should decide what would be the ideal situation, evaluate the current situation, and identify those factors which will motivate change and those which will resist change. The factors promoting change are important to identify but they are likely to be less significant than the factors which resist change. The box gives an example of the considerations concerned in increasing cervical cytology uptake.

Implementing change

Managing change consists of minimising the resisting factors and promoting the motivating factors. It is therefore important to identify these as fully as possible before proposing solutions. Once a problem has been identified it is easy to opt for an immediate solution.

Example 2

Before the new contract a practice was considering how it would cope with the increased workload concerned in visiting patients over 75. One option put forward was to appoint an additional practice nurse. An audit of the work involved, however, showed that it could easily be managed by the existing practice nurse together with the doctors.

Discussion Each solution to a problem needs to be evaluated in terms of costs and benefits. These may not be just monetary costs but also time and energy. Sometimes the risks concerned in implementing the change would be too high and the project may need to be temporarily postponed, as shown by the following example.

Example 3

A seven doctor practice employed a senior receptionist who was responsible for much of the practice administration. It became clear that the practice was running inefficiently through lack of managerial skills. The senior receptionist was also registered with the practice as a patient. Although the partners felt that they needed a practice manager, they thought that the effect on the senior receptionist would

19

Important points for managing change

- The broad aims of the practice need to be defined
- A framework that covers the individual components of general practice should be adapted for setting objectives
- Practice staff are more likely to be committed to changes if they are involved in the decisions
- Consultation must ensure that all staff fully understand new processes
- In managing change the resisting factors should be minimised and the motivating factors promoted
- There are various strategies for dealing with human resistance to change

disrupt the practice and decided to postpone the implementation of a manager until the receptionist retired in two years' time.

Discussion   Whenever change is made the new way or working often requires investment of time and energy. If the energy in a practice is being consumed elsewhere, such as coping with imposed change or through personality clashes, the new system may be rejected or not be implemented. It may be prudent to recognise that the change needs to be made but that the present time is wrong.

Dealing with resistance to change

When the task force has decided the most effective way of reaching the defined object not only will it then plan the change programme, it will also need to address the problem of human resistance to change. Change will be threatening for many people in the practice for many reasons, and unless it is dealt with the change process may be delayed, diluted, or even founder.

For any change project resistance may come from a variety of sources and present itself in many forms. Typical forms of human resistance are parochial self interest, misunderstanding and lack of trust, different assessments of the situation and the proposed solution of it, and low tolerance of change.[3] The important thing is to identify the type of resistance which is likely to be met, then to select a strategy for dealing with it. The sort of strategies which could be employed are education and communication, participation and involvement, facili-

Methods for dealing with resistance to change

Approach	Commonly used in situations	Advantages	Drawbacks
Education and communication	Where there is a lack of information or inaccurate information and analysis	Once persuaded people will often help with the implementation of the change	Can be very time consuming if lots of people are involved
Participation and involvement	Where the initiators do not have all the information they need to design the change, and where others have considerable power to resist	People who participate will be committed to implementing change and any relevant information they have will be integrated into the change plan	Can be very time consuming if participants design an inappropriate change
Facilitation and support	Where people are resisting because of adjustment problems	No other approach works as well with adjustment problems	Can be time consuming and expensive and still fail
Negotiation and agreement	Where someone or some group will clearly lose out in a change, and where that person or group has considerable power	Sometimes it is a relatively easy way to avoid major resistance	Can be too expensive in many cases if it alerts others to negotiate for compliance
Manipulation and cooptation	Where other tactics will not work or are too expensive	It can be a relatively quick and inexpensive solution to resistance problems	Can lead to future problems if people feel manipulated

tation and support, negotiation and agreement, manipulation and cooptation, and explicit or implicit coercions.[3] Not all strategies are appropriate for addressing a particular form of resistance, each having their advantages and disadvantages, and some may not be ethically defensible for a particular task force. The box identifies methods for dealing with resistance to change and the situations in which they are commonly used, together with their advantages and disadvantages, the disadvantages often being to do with the pace of change.

Resistance can come from staff, partners, patients, even the family health services authority. The important thing is that it is identified as early as possible, even anticipated. It can then be dealt with as part of the management of the change process, as illustrated by the next example.

Example 4

A partnership of four doctors was considering upgrading their computer system. Three of the partners had entered the practice within the previous seven years, but the senior partner was considering retiring within five years. The initial proposal was rejected by the senior partner, who could see considerable additional work without much benefit. The younger partners reconsidered the problem and offered to undertake much of the additional work, thus resulting in an acceptable solution.

Follow through

When the proposals have been accepted by every member of the practice the new system can be introduced. The introduction needs to proceed at an acceptable pace—too slow and the task force may become impatient, too fast and the implementers become stressed. In planning a time scale it helps to consider the midpoint of the project and set a target date.

Example 5

A five doctor practice wanted to introduce a diabetic clinic; the whole project seemed daunting. A mid-point was determined, a protocol was agreed, equipment was in place, and staff were trained. This was achieved within nine months and the first patients were soon being diverted to the clinic for their care.

Assessment   The task force has a responsibility to assess the impact of the new system, to make sure that it is running smoothly and that minor modifications are made easily. An end point should be identified and although the task force may retain a special interest, it has completed its task.

Conclusion

When introducing change it is important to plan carefully, set achievable targets with clearly defined time limits, communicate throughout the project, listen for rejection, and award praise when success is achieved.

1 Plant R. *Managing change and making it stick.* London: Fontana/Collins, 1987.
2 Royal College of General Practitioners. *What sort of doctor—assessing quality in general practice.* Devon: RCGP, 1984. (Report from general practice 23.)
3 Kotter JP, Schlesinger LA. Choosing strategies for change. In: Mayon White B, ed. *Planning and managing change.* London: Harper and Row, 1979.

Imposed change in general practice

MAIRI G B SCOTT, MARSHALL MARINKER

In the summer of 1989 the government published its intentions for the reform of the NHS, and for a new contract with general practitioners. Both the reforms and the contract were immediately subject to a host of detailed criticisms about content. But behind these criticisms there lay another — that the government was imposing the changes.

All change gives rise to two reciprocal anxieties. Abandoning established habits and arrangements and embracing new ones produce the anxiety of loss and the anxiety of the unfamiliar. In this chapter we are concerned not with the content of change but with its processes. Although we take as our starting point the concerns occasioned by the reforms of the NHS in the past three years, we do so in order to highlight the problems which can arise within each general practice when change is envisaged. These problems are magnified when there is a sense of imposition, of being the victim and not the agent of change.

This sense of imposition seems to relate to four factors: firstly, the degree to which the reasons for change seem to be arbitrary; secondly, the strength of the evidence of the need for change; thirdly, the degree to which the changes are expressed in terms of desired behaviours as opposed to desired outcomes; and, fourthly, the choice of strategies used to effect the change. We examine these factors in detail below.

Reasons for change

For the most part in general practice the reasons for change seem to be accidental. That is to say they seem to be a part of what may be described as the natural development of a practice. Even when they take place suddenly or unexpectedly they are accepted because the reasons are perceived to be inevitable—the product of human vagaries. There may be shifts in the local population, perhaps the proportion of elderly people has increased over the years; patterns of morbidity may change, sometimes abruptly; there may be staff related problems—partners quarrel, become ill, or resign; the practice may be invited to start vocational training; and so on. Such reasons for change may be burdensome but they will be perceived as accidental. They will certainly pose difficult problems but they will not be seen as having been arbitrarily imposed.

When change is perceived as having been willed by others rather than occasioned by need there is a sense of arbitrariness. The new contract, again, is the most obvious recent example. It was the sense that activities were willed as a matter of policy, politically decided and enforced by a monopolistic employer or commissioner, that caused the sense of helplessness and hopelessness.

It is not only governments that can engender these negative feelings. They can and often do arise within partnerships and group practices. A precedent partner arbitrarily decides to change his half day, or blocks the use of a deputising service, or persistently frustrates the wish of the others to employ additional staff. Change seems to be arbitrary when the initiator is strong and the evidence of need for change is weak.

Points to note

- Change necessitated by circumstances is acceptable in general practice
- Change willed and enforced by others is considered arbitrary
- Often evidence is not available for required change
- Change based on fashion is less acceptable than that based on sound evidence
- Imposed change is more acceptable if it is expressed in terms of outcome rather than detailed behaviour
- The positive way to deal with imposed change is to create a sense of ownership of the change within the practice

---

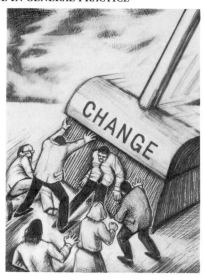

Evidence of the need for change

It would be comforting if all the changes required in general practice were based on reliable evidence from good empirical research. In the case of the new general practitioners' contract the evidence was either lacking or pointed in directions quite different from those proposed by the contract.[1] Often, however, the evidence is simply not available, or is confused. We would argue, for example, that even in the absence of hard evidence counselling reduces morbidity or improves prognosis; counselling remains valuable because of what it says about the humane intentions of medical care.[2] The practice of medicine cannot be driven by the evidence and rules of scientific inquiry alone. The doctor is not a clinical experimenter, but a healer. It is not only the provenance of change that is important but the openness with which that provenance is disclosed and discussed.

Change based on the vagaries of fashion is much less persuasive than change based on sound evidence. Fashion has played an important part in the development of twentieth century general practice. For the past 20 years primary care team work, educationalism (including role play and video consultation analysis), screening, health promotion, and performance review have all been fashionable. Although each of them has enhanced the character and complexity of modern British general practice, they were first and foremost fashions, with relatively short life spans. Most of them were driven by a small number of proselytising advocates (indeed one of us cannot be exonerated from much of this). In so far as the spread of the fashion has been experienced as growth and enlightenment, the changes were acceptable. But there remains the sense of being a slave to fashion. The violence of that term may explain much of the resentment and disdain expressed by general practitioners for the relatively innocent enthusiasms of academic bodies like the Royal College of General Practitioners.

Processes and goals

The creation of health promotion clinics, and in particular the introduction of protocols for these clinics, is an example of change not in the goals of care but in the detailed processes. To predict the activities of doctors' consultations as part of a contract is to rob them of their professionalism. It reduces the practice of medicine to a form of art which is no more creative or responsive than painting by numbers. This contrasts considerably with the implementation of change concerned not with processes but goals, as shown in the following example.

Example

The practice has discovered that its appointment book has become increasingly filled, that patients are unable to see the doctor of their choice within a reasonable period of time, and the number of "extras" at each surgery grows from month to month. The change required is an improvement in the accessibility of the doctors.

Consider the number of possible options. It may be necessary to increase the number of consulting hours each week. This may entail the reallocation not only of time but also of space. The practice may have reached the point when an additional doctor or nurse should be introduced. The problem may be solved by creating fixed hours for telephone consultations. Inquiry may disclose that some doctors have very high recall rates, so that less than a third of their consulting slots are available for patients with new problems. The reasons for this can be explored and alternative solutions arrived at. In this example although the goal (better accessibility) may be imposed, the response is a professional one—it allows the professionals to propose solutions and to make choices. A sense of ownership is created.

27

Strategies for effecting change

Leadership

Whether the reasons for change are internal or external to the practice, whether the substance of the change seems to be imposed or not, change cannot be managed without leadership, and leadership is an uncomfortable concept in British general practice. The culture of general practice in this country is fiercely egalitarian. In part this is reflected in a continuing attachment to the independent contractor status within the NHS, even though the advantages of this may have diminished over the years. It is reflected in the model democracy of the BMA and the local medical committees. Within each individual practice partners today rapidly proceed to parity, not only parity of income with other partners who may have been in the practice for 20 years or more, but parity of workload and responsibility. Even when this is manifestly not the case there is a fierce attachment to the appearance of such equity. It is deeply unfashionable today to use the term "senior partner" without shyly indicating that quotation marks have been used.

Leadership in the practice may depend on several factors. There may indeed be a senior partner who exercises leadership on the basis of precedence or assumed authority. Leadership may be charismatic, a combination of enthusiasm, drive, and charm creating its own authority. Leadership may be appointed or delegated. A powerful partner or subgroup may cede power to one of their number. Sometimes the leadership is democratically elected by the group. Finally, leadership may be sapiential, deriving its authority from what it is that the doctor is believed to know and be capable of doing.

If the leadership is insecurely based, if it is only precedent, or charismatic or appointed, the freedom to act will be limited, and the trust of the group will be ungenerously given. If the leadership is more secure, if it represents the will of the majority or is seen to be justified by the competence of the individual, a more robust and creative leadership becomes possible.

Good leadership is the characteristic not of the individual but of the whole group. Without cooperation and consent the leader may produce a sparkling performance yet achieve next to nothing. It is important to remember that leadership is not necessarily a role, stable over time, and common to all the practice's endeavours. More commonly there is an elaborate dance of leadership between the

28

partners, with different individuals assuming the role of leader, in relation to the task to be undertaken and the trust which the group is prepared to give.

When people are motivated to change by the exercise of threats and sanctions, by the calling in of old debts and the striking of new bargains, by rewards that are bribes and explanations which are bluff, the sense of ownership evaporates. Dishonest leadership creates its own sense of imposed change.

Communication

It is a cliche of organisational theory, and of the sociological critique of doctors, that poor communication is the root of most management problems. But poor communication has a variety of causes. It is not simply a consequence of verbal incompetence or incontinence. Failures of communication may occur because of carelessness, conspiracy, or confusion. Most often we fail to communicate because we forget that information is power, and that giving information is empowerment. Failure to communicate can be part of a conspiracy. We fail to communicate or distort the message in order to hide our own mistakes or undeclared intentions. Lastly, and perhaps most commonly, failure to communicate results from confusion, when there seems to be no clear message to transmit. Of course in this situation nothing could be more useful than to communicate the confusion itself. This rarely happens because our medical education has taught us to hide our errors and conceal our ignorance.

Coping with imposed change

The positive response to imposed change is to create a sense of ownership of the change by the practice. It has been a common experience in the wake of the government's new contract that partners and practice teams have been forced to communicate with each other in a new and more helpful way, simply in order to survive the changes. This force majeure enhancement of general practice partnerships may be the most important (if unintended) benefit of the new contract. In response to the contract there has been widespread debate among general practitioners and within partnerships about the goals of good medical care, about what it is that would be worth achieving.

In an open society there is no unreasonable bureaucratic dictat that cannot be circumvented by intelligently misreading the rules. Practices and authorities can agree to aggregate so called health promotion consultations, so as to create fictional but paid health promotion "clinics." Course tutors will categorise courses to satisfy the idiosyncratic demands for different categories in order to qualify for the postgraduate education allowances. A programme concerned with diabetes mellitus can easily be classified as clinical medicine, or as practice management, or as prevention, without changes to its content.

Conclusion

This is the "age of contract." No matter what the political complexion of future governments, the NHS will henceforward be shaped by specific and detailed contracts. The professional staff of the NHS will be accountable for the fulfilment of these contracts, and the practice of medicine will in the future be determined by their content in exactly the same way as the education of doctors is now predicted by our college examinations.

Klein has commented that at the close of the twentieth century the relationship between all the professions and society is changing from one based on status to one based on contract.[3] By "status" we believe that Klein referred not only to social authority but to moral authority and trust. The age of contract holds many attractive possibilities. Tightly constructed contracts may greatly reduce waste, boost efficiency, permit rational planning, and ensure public accountability.

No planned health service can function without attention to the cost of services, to the calculation of cost benefit and opportunity cost, to performance indicators, explicit standards, compliance, conformity, controls, and accountability. These are the characteristics of the age

---

Contracts in the NHS: advantages and disadvantages

- Contracts may reduce waste, improve efficiency, and enable national planning
- Contracts may devalue creativity
- There may be less emphasis on the needs of the individual patient and a preoccupation with group characteristics
- Strong contracts enfeeble professionalism

---

of contract in medicine. They are the inevitable consequences of the growing demand for medical care, the growing success and cost of biotechnology, and the growing friction between desire and expectation on the one hand and financial constraint on the other.

But the age of contract also has its dangers. Too easily contracts can generate a repressive and controlling influence. Compliance can be valued above creativity. The power of numerate evidence from populations can be exaggerated. Medicine can become preoccupied with the characteristics of groups and become distracted from the assessment of, and response to, the needs of the individual. The personal, idiosyncratic, scientific, and moral dimensions of medical care can become subordinated to what authority arbitrarily deems to be the public good. Contracts may diminish the importance of the doctor's judgment about his or her unique patient in favour of predetermined choices—choices based on evidence of effectiveness and efficiency derived from studies of classes of patients and people. Strong contracts enfeeble professionalism.

Imposition is the unacceptable face of contract. Imposed change violates the professionalism of doctors, which derives from the internalising of shared standards of technical and moral behaviour. Creating a sense of ownership of change is the only guarantee that the changes will work to produce real gains in the quality of care.

1 Morrell DC. The role of research in development of organisation and structure of general practice. *BMJ* 1991;302:1313-6.
2 Halmos P. *The faith of the counsellors*. London: Constable, 1965.
3 Klein R. From status to contract: the transformation of the British medical profession? In: *Healthcare provision under financial restraint: a decade of change*. London: Royal Society of Medicine, 1991.

Meetings and chairmanship

F D RICHARD HOBBS, SIR MICHAEL DRURY

Practice meetings play a crucial part in effecting change in general practice by identifying the key objectives for progress, helping create the mechanisms by which such change can take place, and following up the results. Meetings have a role in developing effective teamwork among the partners, among members of the practice staff (attached and ancillary), and even among the practice community. The importance of constructive teamwork cannot be overstated as there is considerable agreement that many of the best examples of primary care are team based,[1][2] a view that has long been supported by government.[3]

It will be all too clear to many practitioners, however, that meetings can also be time consuming and non-constructive, or even destructive. Unsuccessful meetings can therefore actually inhibit team development and the process of change. Factors that help to produce successful meetings include: the setting of clear objectives for the meeting; a membership that represents everyone with a stake in these objectives; enabling participation during the meeting; reaching clear decisions and reviewing subsequent progress; seeking times and venues for meetings that are achievable for most members; and good chairmanship.

Setting clear objectives and membership

Objectives need to be considered early, reviewed repeatedly, and made clear to members. Such task setting will initially help to determine the composition of the membership. For example, doctors' workload or practice finance meetings might require only partners and the practice manager, but most clinical meetings will require broad representation of doctors, nurses, and administrative staff. Ideally, everyone who has a role in the topics to be discussed should be involved.

In large practices with many attached staff this might mean that representatives of interest groups are chosen to attend most of the meetings, if the membership is to be kept to a manageable size. It is often held that the effectiveness of a meeting is inversely related to the number of people present, although a balance needs to be struck between keeping the size small and achieving adequate coverage. If representatives are chosen this may require that the group represented has a separate opportunity to debate the issues in order that decisions can be seen to be part of team activity. Furthermore, there should always be some opportunity, even if it is only an annual meeting, for all individuals to attend a practice meeting with an agenda that covers relevant issues with a section for any other business.

Adopting this approach to meetings will inevitably lead to allocating separate tasks to different subgroups who have their own dedicated series of discussions. This does not mean that ever more time is spent on talking as subgroups will meet at differing intervals and for different times. Furthermore, if meetings are successful in achieving effective change this will lead to more efficient use of time elsewhere with a consequent improvement of motivation and self esteem.

Enabling participation and reaching decisions

Practice members are more likely to get involved if they believe the issue to be of personal relevance. For this reason the topics debated in practice meetings will often include frequently recurring issues, such as organisational problems—not enough appointments, staff grievances, lack of equipment—and patient problems—such as abusive

---

- Meetings are crucial for identifying a practice's objectives
- Meetings encourage teamwork

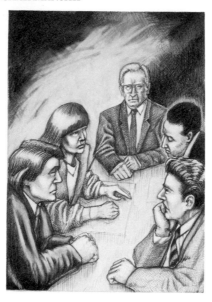

patients, wheelchair access, children in waiting rooms. These sorts of difficulties must be debated, solutions identified, and action taken. Avoidance of the issues will inevitably lead to staff or patient disaffection. If they are recurring problems they need recurring attention.

Another way of organising a meeting is to orient it around a specific task, where improving the quality of care of a particular group of patients (such as diabetic patients) or a practice activity (such as repeat prescribing) is the sole purpose for the discussions. Task driven meetings have a greater potential for creating real teamwork as many health care workers will feel especially motivated to contribute to a clinical care subject. Certain ingredients, however, are essential if the meetings are to succeed in generating change by staff working together more effectively. These include respect for each member's special skills; support for the team approach; involvement in the negotiation of team objectives; and acceptance of the consensus view. With this approach should come trust and thereby cooperation. A task oriented meeting should therefore promote clinical care that is consistent, with common team objectives and agreed management protocol or plans; efficient, with clearly allocated team roles and responsibilities; and effective, with consensus and audit of care.

A series of meetings that achieves positive results, such as the systematic care of all diabetic patients in the practice, will boost the practice team's confidence in its individual members. This will have beneficial effects on most areas of the practice and should encourage ongoing commitment to the process of planned change.

Reviewing progress

Having made decisions in meetings, the consequences must be reviewed to assess effectiveness and the need for further debate. Such peer referenced audits should reinforce the importance of the meetings and also add an educational component to the content of successful meetings. The review of decisions should stimulate the confidence of the practice in stating its health care objectives unequivocally, such as in its annual report, or by the production of a drug formulary,[4] or clinical protocols,[5][6] or even a practice manifesto.[7]

Times and venues

The time and venue of a meeting may be the most difficult components to effect equitably. Ideally, meetings should be held in convenient locations, which will usually be in the practice. Occasionally, however, it may be appropriate to get away from the practice, especially if major issues are to be discussed—perhaps a yearly meeting at an attractive hotel or conference centre for the purpose of setting annual objectives and reviewing a previous annual report. This could be organised outside the working week, with some social event afterwards if the funding permitted.

Most meetings should be limited to a time considered most convenient to most members. Once running, however, the meeting time and day should remain constant, so that it becomes a routine inclusion in each member's diary. If what is discussed in meetings is deemed relevant and discussion stimulates change, then people will find time to attend and contribute. It is important for people attending a meeting to know when it will begin and end; people drifting in and out will destroy effectiveness.

Chairmanship

Without meetings there will not be common objectives,[8] and this will seriously inhibit teams working for change. However, the components that have been identified as contributing to a successful meeting are heavily dependent on the success of chairmanship. The role of the chairman in meetings has never been quite the same since John Cleese, in the film *Meetings Bloody Meetings* (Video-Arts, London), pictured the nightmare scenario of always finishing up a meeting exactly where it started. Although the experience may be all too familiar, the way out of the quandary is not. He made it apparent that this largely depends on the quality of the chairmanship. The role of the chairman is fourfold: to agree an agenda; to run the meeting to time; to allow opinions to be voiced; and to ensure decisions are made.

The agenda

The agenda has to be agreed in such a way that it includes all the items and yet there is sufficient time for them to be discussed. Part of the agenda will depend on matters arising from the minutes of the previous meeting. It is very important that everything is included for otherwise the section labelled any other business will get out of hand. A trap for the unwary, however, is to allow the debate on items already discussed to be repeated. Generally speaking the matters arising section entails reporting what has happened concerning that item since the previous meeting. Usually a task will have been given to someone relating to the item under discussion and this is when they have to report back. The chairman should then be able to identify the key issue, make a summary, and, if necessary, secure a decision. One

---

Important points about practice meetings

- Everyone who has a role in the topics to be discussed should be involved
- In large practices representatives of interest groups can be chosen to attend
- Task oriented meetings may provide a good option
- Meetings should be held in convenient locations at convenient times
- The success of a meeting depends heavily on the quality of chairmanship
- The length of the agenda is critical
- Everyone should have an opportunity to express their views
- Tasks allocated at a meeting should be carefully minuted and clear instructions sent after the meeting to the people concerned

---

aim should be to try to get that matter resolved so that it ceases to be a running item (or a running sore) on agenda after agenda. Making summaries from time to time is a helpful way to make certain that issues are clear and that the person taking the minutes knows what to record.

The rest of the agenda will consist of new items, usually taken in order of priority so that the most important, and lengthy, items can be dealt with while everyone is there and still alert. The length of the agenda is critical. It must be containable within the time allotted. If there are too many items the chairman must devise another strategy for dealing with the matters so that everyone feels they will be properly attended to in due course. The agenda must be ready in adequate time for people to prepare themselves for the meeting, otherwise a lot of time will eventually be wasted, though there is no guarantee the agenda will be read.

Time

The effective use of time is the hallmark of really good chairmanship. Firstly, it is necessary to decide where you want to be at the end of the meeting; what views must be obtained before the meeting ends; and what decisions must be made. Unless the chairman has a clear view of where he or she wishes to be at say 3 pm it will prove to be impossible to organise the meeting effectively and efficiently. Of course it does not always work out the way it was planned, but if there is no framework the chairman cannot devise a strategy for getting the agenda dealt with. Success entails keeping control over the meeting by allowing people to speak only when they are called in turn, seeing that all present have an opportunity to put their views forward uninterrupted, judging when all the points have been raised, and cutting off repetition, and, finally, extracting a decision. Sometimes the decision is best put to a vote, but generally speaking voting forces people to harden attitudes and thus should be used fairly sparingly. It needs firmness to keep this measure of discipline but it must be done with politeness. The time the chairman has to be really ruthless is when "submeetings" begin around the table. This is the point at which a meeting can disintegrate and offenders should be firmly called to order.

Opinions

At the end of a meeting the participants should feel that they have had an opportunity to voice their views. Attenders seem to be divided between those who have a lengthy view on any subject, often only repeating views already expressed, and those who stay silent through shyness or because they are genuinely undecided and wish to hear different points of view before committing themselves. A sensitive chairman will encourage the shy or undecided members while discouraging those who are too lengthy. Observers of the bedside scene will often note the same technique used on the silent or garrulous patient being transferred quite effectively to the meeting room. The silent members should be asked for their views from time to time and encouraged to feel a sense of ownership in the decisions taken.

Decisions

The objective of a meeting must be to obtain a decision. This does not necessarily mean that the item is finally dealt with but does mean that the next set of actions are decided. Every agenda should conclude with a note describing by whom and when the action is to be taken. This should be carefully minuted and it is a considerable kindness to people to write to them afterwards so they have a clear understanding of what is expected of them. This saves a lot of trouble in the future for the chairman who is trying to keep the momentum going.

Conclusion

The chairman has a pivotal role in setting the atmosphere of meetings. Do members feel welcome? Are their contributions valued? Is their presence or their apology for absence properly noted? If people can be helped to enjoy them they may feel John Cleese's title does not always apply to their meetings.

1 Jarman B, Cumberlege J. Developing primary health care. *BMJ* 1987;**294**:1005-8.
2 Department of Health and Social Security. *Neighbourhood living: a focus for care. Report of the community nursing review.* London: HMSO; 1986.
3 Department of Health and Social Security. *Annual Report 1974.* London: HMSO, 1974.
4 Grant DA, Gregory GB, Zwanenberg TD. Development of a limited formulary for general practice. *Lancet* 1985; i1030-2.
5 Mant D, McKinlay C, Fuller A, Randall T, Fullard E, Muir J. Three year follow up of patients with raised blood pressure identified at health checks in general practice. *BMJ* 1989;**298**:1360-2.
6 Fullard EM, Fowler GH, Gray JAM. Promoting prevention in primary care: controlled trial of low technology, low cost approach. *BMJ* 1987;**294**:1080-2.
7 Adelaide Medical Centre Primary Health Care Team. A primary health care team manifesto. *Br J Gen Prac* 1991;**41**:31-3.
8 Marsh GN, Kaim-Caudal P. *Team care in general practice.* London: Croom Helm, 1976.

Practice managers and practice management

LIN MACMILLAN, MIKE PRINGLE

Practice managers are something of a new breed. They are evolving into serious professionals at breakneck speed with, in many cases, considerable autonomy in running practices—practices which have turnovers similar to small or medium sized businesses.

Knowledge of the NHS and medical work is an advantage, but not essential. Training and experience in management skills is more useful, as these can be adapted to different environments without difficulty if the manager is flexible and willing to learn. One prime skill is that of reacting to, influencing, and modifying change within and outside the practice. In this article we look at the general role of the new practice managers and especially at those skills required in the management of change.

Personal and personnel skills

A successful practice manager will utilise all the wiles of a good general manager of any efficient organisation. Any team needs motivating, and this requires the qualities of leadership. This sounds, and is, nebulous, but leadership involves embodying the common aim of the practice through a constant striving for its agreed objectives. It can, of course, be expressed by many team members, not least in clinical issues by the doctors and nurses. For the practice manager leadership must involve all the practice members in working to perfect the organisation which provides the essential support to a successful consultation.

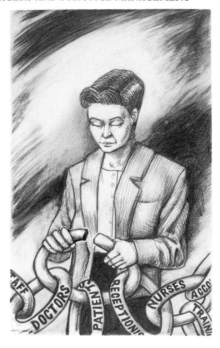

Good leaders are not authoritarian, nor are they shrinking violets. They believe in forging consensus and then helping everybody to share in the implementation. They delegate, with support, and with reasonable expectations of an individual's capabilities. They value people for what they can do and help them to recognise and tackle those areas they find difficult.

The practice manager should be tactful and must have a sense of humour. This is just as essential when dealing with difficult patients who want to see "whoever is in charge" as when dealing with rota clashes between receptionists who all want the same holiday weeks. Many patients are not yet familiar with the role and responsibilities of a practice manager, and some staff members, including doctors, find it difficult to adjust to new hierarchies. The ability to switch concentration from one subject to another quickly is highly desirable, particularly when a crisis occurs. Initiative, ability to work under pressure, and the gift of not being easily flustered are therefore important.

Important skills are required for managing people. Many people feel threatened by change, and a good manager can emphasise the positive points of innovation while helping staff to explore means of dealing with any problems arising. Good communications within the practice and with external bodies need to be established, but this can be extremely difficult. Trying to get everyone together at once can be almost impossible—doctors are on duty and must, of course, put patients' demands before practice meetings, and many ancillary staff are part time and work shifts.[1]

Example 1

One of our practices has solved the problem of communication to some extent by two methods. A regular newsletter is prepared about once a month and is circulated to every member of the practice, from the doctors to the cleaning staff. Important information, changes in procedure, and some light hearted items are all included, and this has gone a long way to preventing the "Nobody told me that" syndrome.

Additionally, a staff representative committee was set up, which meets quarterly. Each area of the practice elected a representative, who collects points for the agenda from his or her colleagues. With the practice manager acting as secretary and one of the doctors chairing the committee, in rotation, ideas can be explored, procedures refined, and problems aired. This acts as a very useful forum, and most of the items raised have been very constructive.

Sharing responsibilities

Having appointed a practice manager, many doctors may find it difficult to adapt. Some are only too delighted to relinquish the burden of administration and concentrate on the clinical aspects of their work. Others may be reluctant to let go the management cloak which they have had to wear in the past. Some may not wish even a

---

Advantages of setting up a staff representative committee

- Communication reaches everyone in the practice
- Everyone can play a part in discussing ideas and problems
- Feedback from staff representative committees can be very useful to the practice manager and the doctors

41

senior member of staff to have knowledge of their income, and so may wish to retain that aspect of the work themselves. Partners with strong personalities may find the process of delegation somewhat unfamiliar and uncomfortable and may find it easier in the short term to retain their control.

Undeniably many doctors have considerable knowledge of "the system." The internal workings of a family health services authority or a district health authority can be mystifying to a novice to general practice, and business management skills are no substitute for a doctor's knowledge and experience of how it all works.

No one can deny, though, that the new general practitioners' contract has meant an indigestible amount of paperwork, and many hours have had to be spent considering how a practice should adapt to the changing requirements of primary health care. Unprecedented hours have had to be given over to training, particularly in those practices using computer systems for the first time, and changes in culture and working methods must be communicated to staff. Many practices have had to set up systems to cope with patient call and recall to achieve target payments, visiting over 75 year olds, three year health checks, and health promotion clinics. Some of these demands have meant investing large sums of money in new equipment; obtaining the best terms from suppliers requires a great deal of time and energy. Where could doctors find the time to address all these areas and continue to see as many patients as ever before? Many practices have already decided that they could not do the impossible, and have therefore sought the services of a professional manager who can devote time to the non-clinical side of running the practice.

Management or administration?

But some practices already had "practice managers" before the new contract. The new style business manager, however, is really a phenomenon of the past two years or so. Before that many people with the title of practice manager were in fact practice administrators.[2] These were often senior receptionists who had worked their way up through the ranks and who had been given the added responsibilities of ensuring that claims were filled in correctly and dispatched on time; that stationery and supplies were ordered when required; and that the staff rota was covered for holidays and sickness. In addition their duties might have included doing the wages and the accounts.

New style practice managers do, or oversee, all of these things, but their remit covers a great deal more besides. Dealing with staff in a wider sense—interviewing, appointing, training, discipline, and appraisals are areas which may previously have been dealt with by the staff partner, or perhaps not dealt with at all. With respect to financial management a practice manager's remit includes wages and salaries, accounts, cash flow analysis, and budget control. In practices where this has always been left to the accountant the involvement of the practice manager may have a beneficial effect on accountancy charges and the practice's understanding of its financial affairs.

Managing change

Development of new or refined procedures to aid the smooth running of the practice is another area where management skills come into play. Firstly, the ideas have to be thought through; secondly, they have to be sold to all members of the practice; and, thirdly, they have to be implemented efficiently and with the minimum amount of friction.

Example 2

One practice had traditionally paid the staff weekly by bank transfer. This meant that the practice manager had to devote about three hours a week to this task—time which could have been better utilised for other work. The idea of monthly payment of staff was first raised by the practice manager in a partnership meeting. The advantage of time saved, coupled with a reduction in bank charges (there would be 12 sets of bank transfers each year as opposed to 52) convinced the partners that this would be a step forward, providing the staff were in agreement.

Each member of staff was then consulted individually by the practice manager and asked if monthly payment would cause them

---

Guidelines for managing change

- Seek consensus on the changes required by consulting widely and individually—identify as many gains for as many people as possible
- Especially value the opinions of those most affected by the changes
- Try to minimise the effects of the change in the transition period

---

any difficulty. Only one had any doubts about the change, but she agreed to abide by the majority decision. To make the transition to monthly payment easier in the first month staff were paid half their monthly salary after two weeks and the remainder at the end of the month.

Future development of the practice manager

As the number of fundholding practices increases the role of the practice manager has the potential to develop even further. An ability to negotiate contracts and the skills to manage the funds efficiently may well be required of many existing practice managers. Negotiating techniques are not, however, restricted to fundholding managers. The role of the family health services authority is now considerably different from that of the old family practitioner committee. A family practitioner committee existed to carry out the administration relating to the providers of primary health care, whereas family health services authorities are now told that they must manage the service. The most effective line of communication between family health services authorities and general practice is often at the management level, but since the implementation of the new contract relations have not always been easy.

So a new style practice manager is often a professional manager, with training and experience at senior level. To some degree they are personnel managers, accounts managers, estates officers, and general

---

Some duties of the practice manager

• To achieve organisation that gives maximum support to consultation

• To deal with non-clinical crises as they occur

• To ensure good communication within the practice and with external bodies such as family health services authorities

• To ensure adequate training of staff to cope with changes such as new computer systems

• Dealing with staff issues, such as interviewing, discipline, and appraisals

• Financial management—that is, dealing with salaries, accounts, cash flow analysis, and budget control

• Developing new procedures and implementing changes

---

managers all rolled into one. Some are being recruited from the world of commerce and industry, but this is not to say that old style practice managers are sent packing. Those who can adapt and take advantage of the increased training opportunities now available are just as likely to succeed as the whizz kids from outside. Such people deserve admiration for the way in which they have been able to embrace the new order.

But once the practice manager is in place, what then? Perhaps all practice managers should take as their motto the words of the British philosopher Alfred North Whitehead, who said, "The art of progress is to preserve order amid change, and to preserve change amid order."

Conclusions

The pace of change in the NHS shows little sign of slowing down in the short term, and this will mean that practices will have to be willing and able to adapt to the adjustments required. A practice which is efficient and financially sound is a great deal more likely to succeed in implementing a new order, and this requires good organisation. All staff will have to have clearly defined roles and a commitment to the practice's objectives and to their own personal goals as part of the team. This will require investment of time and money in staff training to ensure that everyone understands what they are doing, and why, and the necessity for flexibility and cooperation. Practice procedures require scrutiny to ensure that they are logical, easily understood by patients and staff, and are capable of adaptation when unusual circumstances occur.

Planning must play a greater part in the life of a practice than may have been the case in the past. Business plans are now required by many family health services authorities but should in any case be used by every practice to determine the way forward. Short and long term plans covering every aspect of the practice should be developed to facilitate achievement of aims and review of progress. Clear avenues of communication must be laid so that all members of the team are familiar with the practice philosophy.

Doctors who employ practice managers must be prepared to delegate defined areas of authority to them. They must also be clear just what role they see the manager developing within the practice. For this reason every practice manager should have a comprehensive job description detailing all areas of responsibility. Coupled with

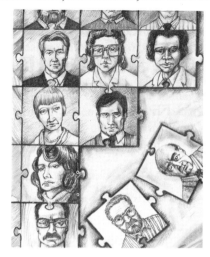

reactions depending on the individual's educational or cultural background. Similarly, the same education given to people of differing culture will result in differing attitudes to change. Why, for instance, does the experience of working under an autocratic and exploitative senior partner lead some general practitioners rigorously to avoid following suit, while others can't wait to assume the senior partner's mantle?

The shortcomings of medical education and training are all too well known. It singularly fails to teach the use of clinical logic to manage uncertainty and that general practice, dealing with initially small variations from normal health without instant recourse to technological investigation, centres on the management of uncertainty, and therefore leaves the alumni with a load of anxiety.

Experience isn't history, it's biography. Of the myriad things that happen to us or which we see happen to others only those which are "internalised"—that is, connected up with our other observations and values—constitute experience. Essentially, therefore, experience as a predictor of response to change or suggested change is to do with feelings, and may not be strictly "rational" or "objective."

The culture of power

But education and experience are not superimposed on a blank sheet. They happen to people who belong to, or come from, a given background, characterised by its values and beliefs: a culture. These values and beliefs are absorbed from our earliest years and are strongly influenced by the community in which we grow up, and therefore by factors such as ethnicity, social class, and local ways of looking at things (for instance, the difference in views between north and south, whether Scandinavian compared with Italian, or Cumbrian compared with Kentish).

Such absorption isn't limited to childhood, and values and beliefs continue to be inculcated as we clamber up the educational ladder. As we do so, the power of precept is displaced by that of example, and role models, negative as well as positive, become strong influences on attitudes and values. The power exercised by senior clinicians and the way they exercise power is perhaps central to their influence as models. The most important aspect of culture with regard to change in general practice is power.

The traditional British system of teaching values, inculcated by the public schools and the forces for which they were preparing people, was that power and privilege had to be earned by taking responsibility (hence the prefect, the junior officer). This method may always have been for a minority of people, and certainly is now, when it seems that power is seen as a desirable end in itself, and responsibility an unfortunate and hopefully avoidable encumbrance. But the practice of medicine starts with responsibility, and to discharge that responsibility you often have to exert power. (In the Larrinaga operating theatre of the old Liverpool Royal Infirmary was a quote from Hippocrates along the lines of "It is the duty of the surgeon to make his assistants and the patient cooperate with him"). Unfortunately in the traditional British culture power, like enthusiasm and cleverness, is deeply suspect, and therefore disguised, so that the exercising of it is often covert, idiosyncratic, and arbitrary.

- Medical education fails to teach the use of clinical logic to manage uncertainty

- Experience as a predictor of response to change is to do with feelings and not strictly objective

- As well as social class and ethnicity doctors' beliefs are shaped by their role models throughout their training, and these will influence their response to change

The value of respect

Over and over again in these chapters the question of relationships within hierarchies, whether between partners or between principals and other members of staff has come up but seldom been addressed in cultural terms, and, in particular in terms of the culture of power. In any organisation who has power over whom, and what sort of power, and how it is exerted, are crucial factors in the way the organisation works. Does seniority confer power; if it does, why, and what sort of power; and is this generally accepted within the practice? These things are unlikely to have been dealt with explicitly. Are staff colleagues, subordinates, or servants (in reality if not in name)? Useful evidence is the use of first names, nicknames, or titles.

The abuse of power can and does obstruct growth and desirable change, but growth and change can be achieved only by the proper exercising of power. Management training, good chairmanship, well organised meetings, force field analysis, Belbin inventories, and all the rest of the important tools discussed in this series will be of little avail if the existence of power is dishonestly concealed, if it is arrogated rather than awarded (sapiential leadership), or if it is used capriciously. It has to be faced that organisations, including practices, are not democracies: power is not evenly distributed (any more than rewards), and the pretence that it is can lead to disillusionment and resentment when the chips are down.

What must be evenly distributed is respect: everybody who does his or her job properly is entitled to the wholehearted respect of every other member of the practice. A person who knows that he or she has the respect of colleagues has the personal space to cope with change. Someone who feels undervalued has to rely on self esteem, which is tied up with day to day activities. If the tea lady feels she is the only person who realises how much she is needed and how carefully she makes and presents the vital fluid, she is unlikely to welcome the introduction of a vending machine so as to free her to take on other responsibilities.

Differences in social class

Unfortunately another characteristic of British culture is its subtle and pervasive class consciousness. Not only power, but personal space and the right to respect vary with status on the many runged ladder of perceived class. But just as power is too uncomfortable a concept in this culture to be dealt with openly and honestly so is class consciousness. Other cultures from which many general practitioners come, have wider class differences and different ways of handling them. As a result relationships within hierarchies are likely to be coloured by subliminal feelings about class and therefore worth.

To understand the interaction between education and culture as predictors of reaction to and ability to cope with or manage change we have only to think of students' observations of life on the wards and the behaviour of their role models there. Students from middle class backgrounds are likely to accept the exercising of power and perfunctory courtesy towards others exhibited by some consultants as desirable features in their role models, while those from more disadvantaged and politically angry backgrounds may draw exactly opposite conclusions. Both sets of attitudes will colour their subsequent behaviour.

Heterogeneities of general practice

Politicians, civil servants, and managers regard the heterogeneity of general practice as a bad thing, and a challenge to their skills in imposing change. The important thing is for them to differentiate between the heterogeneity that stems from the negative effects of the education, experience, and culture triangle of forces, which is a legitimate target for change towards homogeneity, and that which represents responsiveness to local needs and wants. Furthermore, they should be careful about the criteria by which they choose to define the pattern of practice towards which they wish to move. At first sight these may centre on the features of highly organised practices with computerised systems and training facilities, in purpose built premises with regular team meetings, etc, and decry the single handed practitioner in shabby surroundings. This range of general practitioners might, however, conceal another—from authoritarian doctors who impose the college model in which everyone must toe the line, including patients, to those who provide responsive and sensitive care, who have reacted against regimentation and stayed in the urban jungle because that's where his or her patients felt comfortable.

General practitioners are highly defensive: they still believe that general practice is seen as second class medicine; NHS high brass often talk about it as if it were outside the NHS. At the interface between the NHS and people's health care needs and between

51

primary and secondary care general practice has had no choice but to accommodate to enormous change in needs, the way they are presented, and the technology with which they are met. "Conservatism" in some practices may represent a desperate attempt to hang on to something in a maelstrom of change. (McMillan and Pringle in their chapter on practice managers quote from Whitehead: "The art of progress is to preserve order amid change, and preserve change amid order.")

Conclusion

If heterogeneity in practice performance and, indeed, in response to these articles reflects different resultant behaviours from the interaction between culture, education, and experience, then there is little to be gained by prescribing ways of coping with change, or initiating it, as if they were applicable to all practices and all practitioners. General practitioners and their colleagues will cope with change better if they start by reviewing, honestly and openly, the distribution of power and respect within their partnerships and practices. This is always difficult and often painful: it takes time and is a very private activity. To try to impose it from outside would be counterproductive. Family health services authorities must take this on board and try to work "with the grain."

Partners in
Practice

The primary health care team: history and contractual farces

JOHN HASLER

It is not possible to state precisely when the concept of a team in primary health care became a reality. As with so many developments its progress was slow and its start unrecognisable. Before the arrival of the NHS in 1948 most general practitioners were in single handed practice, often with their wives as their only support—receptionists as such were uncommon. There were no attachments of district nurses and most doctors practised from their own houses.[1] While there had been occasional ideas about a more progressive approach to primary medical care, these had been sporadic and had had little general effect. General practitioners saw their role as reactive and their potential role in prevention of disease had not yet dawned on most of them.

In this chapter I examine subsequent developments in three phases: from the inception of the NHS to the doctors' charter in 1966, from then to the new contract in 1990, and the present.

The '50s were difficult times for general practice. Removed from the hospital service and operating in a financial arrangement where any money spent on staff or premises directly reduced their income, many general practitioners looked with some envy on their specialist colleagues as the hospital service and technological advances took shape. But the frustrations had their positive effects, the most notable of which was formation of the College of General Practitioners, which attracted some of the ablest minds of the day. Some of these people turned their thoughts to starting primary care teams. As money was scarce, buildings often inadequate, and the potential of nursing work in general practice largely unrecognised, the theme at this stage largely concerned the attachment of district nurses and health visitors.

Attachment of nursing staff

The first reports of attachment of local authority nursing staff, who were then working in geographical areas under the control of the medical officers of health, appeared in the '50s and early '60s.[2 3] But it was not all plain sailing. It took men of vision to see the possibilities, and Ian McDougall, county medical officer of health for Hampshire, a stalwart enthusiast for attachment schemes, once recalled how he had been accused by some of his colleagues of dismantling their empires.

Many general practitioners were equally wary of the new developments. In a survey carried out by the Wessex Regional Hospital Board in 1964 less than half of general practitioners wanted health visitors

---

History of the practice team

Before 1948
● General practitioners usually worked singlehandedly

1948-66
● Formation of the College of Practitioners encouraged able thinkers to advocate a team approach in primary care

● The first local authority nursing attachments were made in the 1950s, but many medical officers and general practitioners were wary.

1966-90
● The 1966 Family Doctors' Charter enabled employment of practice staff—70% of the costs were reimbursed

● The role of practice nurses expanded and their number increased

● Practice managers were employed to help with management and administration

● An increasing number of other health care professionals became involved in primary care

1990 onwards
● The workload created by the new general practitioner contract has increased the need for practice nurses and practice managers with proved managerial skills. As their roles expand these members will have a higher profile and may become partners or members of executive boards

---

attached, and this fraction was as low as a quarter in another survey in the previous year conducted by the medical care research unit of Manchester University.[4] One of the problems was that many general practitioners were not entirely clear what health visitors did and, furthermore, in a survey conducted by the Royal College of General Practitioners only a minority of doctors were interested in prevention.[4] In a survey in 1966 nearly half the doctors had difficulty in contacting district nurses and most doctors were ignorant about district nurses' qualifications and the help they could give.[5] By the middle of the '60s it was becoming clear that although the new developments in teamwork were beginning to be accepted, something much more radical was needed if real progress was to be made.

1966-90

The 1966 Family Doctors' Charter provided the contractual framework within which many of the new ideas circulating in general practice could take effect. It stimulated the development of new, larger buildings and made employment of staff by general practitioners a realistic option because 70% of their cost was reimbursed. The number of receptionists and secretaries began to increase. The most important development, however, was the employment of nurses.

Practice nurses

There were two reasons why the employment of nurses was an obvious step in the evolution of primary health care. The first was that in many practices (including those considered relatively advanced in the mid-'60s) most routine nursing work on the premises was done by the doctors: this included giving injections, performing venepuncture, and applying dressings. It made no sense at all to continue in this way. The second reason was that in the mid-'60s, when there was a sporadic development of attachment of district nurses and health visitors, even in practices that had district nurses there were limits within which they had to operate. The number of district nurses who worked in practices and health centres was always limited, and still is today.

Most publications at the time were concerned with routine nursing procedures,[6][7] although two papers in the late '60s described nurses carrying out assessment visits to patients requesting a visit by a doctor,[7][8] an idea which never really caught on, especially as the number

ments reflected developments from the previous decades, such as the concept of health promotion activities.

The new contract importantly did not interfere with the principle that although the general practitioner was responsible for ensuring that the contract was fulfilled, any work considered appropriate could be delegated to others, whether or not they were employed by the doctor. Thus the concept of teamwork was retained. However, the guarantee of 70% reimbursement for all staff up to a ceiling amount was removed, creating a measure of uncertainty for the future.

But the contract had other effects. Much of the new work, such as new registration, three yearly health checks, and health checks for those over 75 and the payment for special clinics stimulated further increases in the number of practice nurses. The new paperwork, especially in fundholding practices, encouraged practices to employ new administrative staff: some practice manager posts were advertised at a salary of over £20 000 a year. A book on practice management was into its second edition within 18 months[19] and another had received orders in excess of 1500 even before it was published.[20]

The future

Already there are some clear questions about the future for primary health care teams.

Nurses

The primary health team has always had a highly complicated managerial structure, chiefly because the attached members are employed not only by an external body but one which, in England and Wales, is not the authority responsible for contracting with the doctors. Furthermore, the fact that some family health services authorities will not pay for clinic sessions done by attached staff has put pressure on some practices to substitute practice nurses for attached nurses, creating frustration and anxieties for attached nurses. There is already a debate about whether attached staff should be employed by the family health services authorities or, even more widely, by general practitioners.[21] Clearly if general practitioners employed the attached staff roles and boundaries would be looked at anew. More delegation of work by doctors is virtually certain, especially regarding prevention and supervision of patients with chronic disease.

Management

Many practice managers are still only administrators, but the new breed of manager is more skilled and has higher expectations. Some practices are already exploring ways in which managers (and nurses) can become partners or members of executive boards. Because of their central role in primary care practice managers are now routinely members of the visiting teams who approve training practices in the Oxford region.

Fundholding has enabled practices to buy in the services of other health care professionals such as physiotherapists and psychologists.

Conclusion

In the end what makes a successful team is not merely the quality of the individual members but how they work together. In recent years an increasing number of educational activities have been devised to promote effective teamwork, and many groups now organise whole days away from the practice, when they can share aims and devise better ways of working together. The potential for new ways of delivering primary care has never been greater.

1 Kuenssberg EV. *The team in primary care. Royal College of General Practitioners members' reference book.* London: RCGP, 1991.
2 Pinsent RJFH, Pike LA, Morgan RH, Mansell JM. The health visitor in a general practice. *BMJ* 1961;suppl 1:123-7.
3 Swift G, McDougall IA. The family doctor and the family nurse. *BMJ* 1964;i:1697.
4 Royal College of General Practitioners. *Present state and future needs. Reports from general practice II.* London: RCGP, 1965:40-3.
5 Hockey L. *Feeling the pulse. Queens Institute of District Nursing Course.* London: Queens Institute of District Nursing, 1966.
6 Marsh GN. Group practice nurse: an analysis and comment on six months' work. *BMJ* 1967:1; 489-91.
7 Hasler JC, Hemphill PMR, Stewart TI, Boyle N, Harris A, Palmer E. Development of the nursing section of the community health team. *BMJ* 1968;iii:734.
8 Weston Smith J, Mottram EM. Extended use of nursing services in general practice. *BMJ* 1967;iv:672.
9 Hasler JC, Greenland AS, Jacka SM, Pritchard PMM, Reedy BELC. Training for the treatment room sister in general practice. *BMJ* 1972;i:232-4.
10 Jacka SM, Griffiths DG. *Treatment room nursing.* Oxford: Blackwell Scientific Publications, 1976.
11 Fowler G, Fullard E, Gray JAM. The extended role of practice nurses in preventive health care. In: Bowling A, Stillwell B, eds. *The nurse in family practice.* London: Scutari, 1988.
12 Marsh GN. *Efficient care in general practice. Oxford GP series 21.* Oxford: Oxford University Press, 1991:11.
13 Thorn PA, Russell RG. Diabetic clinics today and tomorrow: mini clinics in general practice. *BMJ* 1973;ii:534-6.
14 Mackinnon M, Wilson RM, Hardisty CA, Ward JD. Novel role for specialist nurses in managing diabetes in the community. *BMJ* 1989;**299**:552-4.
15 Marsh GN. *Efficient care in general practice. Oxford GP series 21.* Oxford: Oxford University Press, 1991:40-51.

16 Pearson R. Asthma care in general practice. Stratford-upon-Avon: Asthma Society Training Centre, 1988.
17 Anderson SA, Hasler JC. The effects of counselling in general practice. *J R Coll Gen Pract* 1979;**29**:352-6.
18 Pritchard P. Patient participation in general practice. *J R Coll Gen Pract [Occas Pap]* 1981:**17**.
19 Drury VWM, ed. *The new practice manager*. Oxford: Radcliffe Medical Press, 1990.
20 Hasler JC, Hobden-Clarke L, Bryceland C, Rose P. *Handbook of practice management*. Edinburgh: Churchill Livingstone, 1991.
21 Salisbury C. Working in partnership with nurses. *Br J Gen Prac* 1991;**41**:398-9.

The clinical task

JANET SHEPPARD

In most practices the practice nurse is now an established member of the primary health care team, but this is a relatively new phenomenon. Any attempt to establish when practice nursing began is fraught with difficulty as there is an inevitable discrepancy between the official information and the experience of those who have worked in general practice without an official title or recognition. It is well known that the general practitioner's wife who had nursing qualifications was called on to use her bandaging and other nursing skills in between acting as receptionist, nanny, and chief cook and bottle washer to her overworked husband; and it may reasonably be supposed that the nursing duties were a forerunner to practice nursing as it is today.

Development of practice nursing

The chief factor in bringing about the change in practice nursing was the revision of general practitioners' terms of service in the mid-1960s, which not only introduced a 70% subsidy for employing a nurse in the practice but also specifically encouraged general practitioners to delegate tasks to nurses with the proviso that "reasonable steps are taken to ensure continuity of treatment . . ." and that the member of staff to whom such tasks were delegated was ". . . competent to carry out such treatment."[1]

In 1968 the Health Service and Public Health Act allowed district nurses to treat patients in practice premises as well as in their own

63

homes, opening the door for delegation of tasks to a wider client base. It rapidly became clear, however, that district nursing staff had insufficient time to take on this new role without compromising their domiciliary work. The door had been opened a crack, and it seems there were plenty of nurses waiting outside to push it open wider.

Department of Health figures indicate that in 1977 there were about 1500 practice nurses employed under the ancillary staff scheme. By 1984 the figure had reached 2000 whole time equivalents in England and Wales, and by 1986 it was 3700[2]; and with increasing numbers of nurses employed by local district health authorities to work in general practice the nurse was clearly an important part of the primary health care team. By 1988 the figure had doubled, and, with the advent of the new general practitioners' contract, by the end of 1991 there were about 18 000 practice nurses in post.

Strength in numbers alone is not sufficient to guarantee success, and those who work in unsatisfactory situations will find scant comfort in knowing they are not alone. To those nurses who feel isolated in their posts, unsupported, and perhaps misunderstood by their employing general practitioners it is only too evident that a disparate group of people who are working under one roof with the same group of patients do not become a team simply by being called one. However, nurses must ensure that they are suitably prepared for their delegated tasks. While there are nurses spending time carrying out

---

Tasks included in the developing role of the practice nurse

- Promotion of self care
- Follow up care after minor surgery in the practice
- Performing immunisations
- Giving vaccinations for foreign travel and advice on health care abroad
- Care of patients with chronic disease in the community
- Performing venepuncture
- Syringing ears
- Taking cervical smears
- The possibility of prescribing by nurses in the future
- Audit and self assessment

tasks for which they have neither been trained nor employed (for example, dispensing) and general practitioners who remain unaware and unconcerned about the potential and limitations of practice nurses, for some practices real teamwork will be nothing more than an interesting theory expounded in erudite medical journals.

Workload of the primary health care team

The 20 year period of growth in practice nursing has also seen considerable change in the workload and structure of the primary health care teams. Indeed there can be few "new" branches of a profession that have seen so many changes in their short life. Changes have occurred in response both to patients' (or clients') expectations and to government moves. It is perhaps fanciful to suggest that no aspect of life is deemed outside the scope of some member of the team. It is certainly true, however, that there is now a much greater emphasis on services provided to "the well." The promotion of self care is now deemed much more important than in the early days of the nurse in general practice, when the members of the team were all concerned with the sick and their families in either a supporting or remedial role.

One outcome of the transfer of patients to the community from institutions for mentally ill and handicapped people and earlier discharge from hospitals has been a blurring of the edges of the roles, and indeed the definitions, of primary health care and community care. The workload of both has increased and a jealously guarded territorial approach can no longer be countenanced.

Role of the practice nurse

The workload of all team members includes considerable time spent treating patients with acute conditions, and the delegation of tasks such as changing dressings and removing sutures after trauma or surgery to the nurse is not a new phenomenon. This delegation has greatly increased, however, as general practitioners have undertaken emergency and minor surgery work in the practice which would previously have been done in hospital. The nursing tasks for such cases are now divided between the practice and district nurses on the basis of the patients' ability to attend the surgery. The presence of a practice nurse has also led to a change in self referral of patients both for treatment and for advice. In some instances the health visitor may previously have been seen as the person most appropriate to under-

65

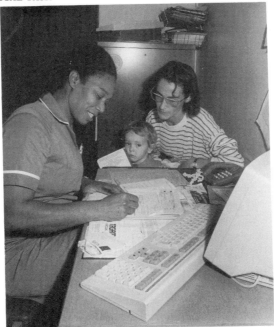

The practice nurse is potentially always available to give treatment or advice

take this role. It should now be recognised that, provided adequate training has been undertaken, the practice nurse can make a valuable contribution in support of the health visitor and district nurse and is potentially always available to meet the demands of today's "instant" society.

Immunisations

There has also been a movement towards the practice nurse performing immunisations. Targets for childhood immunisation are best met by an organised and consistent team approach, with all parties committed to maximum uptake. The health visitor's initial visit to the infant may be the beginning of the process, with the message reinforced by the general practitioner at the six or eight weeks' check. A combined clinic with the health visitor and general practitioner present to monitor progress and give support and advice as necessary and the practice nurse giving the immunisations may well be the most effective way of providing this service. Opportunistic immunisation of non-attenders at the clinic when they attend the practice can be carried out by the practice nurse. Adult immunisation and giving vaccinations for foreign travel and advice on health care abroad are now commonly delegated to practice nurses, enabling a flexible service.

Move to community care

Perhaps the greatest change for the primary health care team in recent years has occurred in the management of chronic diseases. For people with diabetes, asthma, or hypertension the pattern of diagnosis—hospital referral and outpatient follow up, with the general practitioner prescribing drugs and giving support between visits—has been broken, and care in the community has become the norm for all but the most complex cases. For most patients at the very least this is considerably more convenient, and at best they receive personally tailored, systematic care locally from professionals with whom they already have a rapport and in whom they have confidence. Sadly this confidence is sometimes misplaced, as the introduction of payment for health promotion clinics has been responsible for "road to Damascus" experiences for some general practitioners who were previously unwilling to delegate such work to practice nurses, unhappy with the extension of their role beyond anything but task orientated handmaiden.

The move to community care has also given scope for enthusiastic but untrained and unaware nurses to take on roles for which they have had no suitable preparation, and the inevitable loser is the patient. A golden opportunity to review the care of patients with chronic diseases in a team setting, with each team member taking advantage of further training and development and sharing in the drawing up of protocols, has in too many cases been lost. In the best provided for centres, however, there will be access to a community dietician, physiotherapist, chiropodist, and social worker, with referrals made directly by the general practitioner, health visitor, district nurse, and practice nurse.

Accountability

But how have these changes affected those who are providing the care? For the general practitioners there are not only the issues of keeping themselves updated in all aspects of care for all conditions,

67

issues which affect all of the members of the primary health care team, but there is the added concern of clinical responsibility. If general practitioners are to delegate specific tasks to other members of the team they must do so with a clear knowledge of their fellow professionals' capabilities, a knowledge which includes awareness of the content of the training they have undertaken, so that there is no ambiguity about the limitations as well as the extent to which their role can reasonably be extended. Also, all parties concerned must recognise that tasks should be delegated or undertaken only by agreement, with an acknowledgment of individual accountability and where this begins and ends. Professional indemnity is relevant to all concerned, and the terms under which this is applicable are unambiguous and immutable. A nurse undertaking responsibilities for which she has not been trained and assessed as competent is not protected, and no amount of goodwill from her employer will alter this fact.

Communication is a fundamental part of the processes of both delegation and role extension, and there need be no barrier to developing the role of the practice nurse if this is mutually respected. The evidence that this is both possible and successful is widespread, and the Georgian Research Society's pilot study of general practitioners' attitudes towards practice nurses suggests that most practitioners favour the extension of the nurses' role.[3] It has even been suggested more recently that an increase in the number of nurse practitioners could, in conjunction with optimum participation by all members of the primary health care team, enable practitioners to increase their list size relatively painlessly.[4] (Self referral by the patient to a nurse practitioner for diagnosis and treatment of certain conditions to an agreed medical protocol, with referral to the general practitioner of those outside this protocol, is now the chief difference between the nurse practitioner and the practice nurse, and there is obviously scope for developing this role to the benefit of all concerned.)

Prescribing by nurses

The issue of nurse prescribing looks set to rumble on for some time. This should allow all parties concerned to examine the issues carefully as such a radical move raises at least as many questions as it answers. The practice of nurses selecting and administering a treatment (such as applying a dressing) but requiring a general practitioner's signature on the prescription form may be seen as demeaning,[5] and prescribing by nurses would promote greater professional independence in this respect. But accountability issues remain, and there is a need for a considerable training and education programme for those nurses for whom prescribing is proposed. Few nurses currently in post will be equipped for this without a great deal of support, and it is not surprising that employing general practitioners have reservations. Before prescribing is undertaken by nurses it could be beneficial to all parties to discuss aims and objectives, and a locally devised protocol and limited list would ensure that everyone concerned may embark on this new development with confidence.

Audit

This system of evaluation can be effectively applied in other spheres of activity, and indeed audit is a requirement for general practice. This seems entirely reasonable and is an integral part of improving the service and quality of care offered to patients. Audit is most effective if it is undertaken by individual members of the primary health care team, with regular feedback in both directions. Unfortunately it does not come easily to everyone. As many of us trained in an atmosphere where initiative was frowned on, and our work was principally task orientated, the tasks being laid down by the consultant or tradition, it is perhaps understandable that the prospect of self motivation and assessment is a daunting one. Audit need not, however, be seen as a negative and potentially threatening activity. Indeed, it is encouraging to be able to demonstrate both to yourself and to other team members that aims and objectives have been achieved, or that change has begun to take place, and if audit is regularly undertaken any inefficient procedures and systems can be amended before they become too deeply ingrained.

For practice nurses working with team members who are unsure about extension of the nurse's role audit presents an excellent opportunity for nurses to show how successful their position is. Nurses are particularly good at organising, and the organisation of accurate records is fundamental to the audit process. Team audit and feedback may lead to redistribution of tasks and reassessment of systems, and with a cohesive team approach this can only be beneficial, not only in terms of professional development for the team members but most importantly for the patients.

1 Statutory Instrument 1966 No 1210. NHS Eng & Wales Gen Med & Pharm Serv. Reg. 1966.
2 Department of Health. *Statistics for general medical practice in England and Wales, 1979-89.* London: DoH, 1990.
3 Beaton S, Campbell D, O'Sullivan J, Robinson G, Sedgwick J, Tanner S, *et al.* The attitude of general practitioners towards practice nurses: a pilot study. *Br J Gen Pract* 1991;**41**:19-22.
4 Marsh GN. Caring for larger lists. *BMJ* 1991;**303**:1312-6.
5 Crown JM. *Primary Health Care* 1991;**1**:30.

Attached, detached, or new recruits?

CONSTANCE MARTIN

In 1986 community health services were defined by the Department of Health and Social Security as "front line . . . services provided outside hospitals . . . by community nurses, midwives and health visitors and other professions allied to medicine."[1] The part played by community nursing in those front line services has been shaped by many influences over the years. In this chapter I look at some of them and at where community nursing is bound for in future.

Where has community nursing been?

Up until the 1970s district nurses and health visitors were detached from general practice. They worked from a centre and were employed either directly by the local authority or by an association contracted to the local authority to provide nursing and health visiting services. The service was managed by a superintendent who had community nursing qualifications. But because most of the contact between the service and general practitioners was through the superintendent there was often little direct communication between the general practitioner and the nurse.

As early as the 1950s some health districts had recognised that this could create difficulties and were taking steps to overcome them. By 1965 Oxford health district had attached all its district nurses and health visitors to practices; by early 1970, 75% of health visitors and 68% of district nurses in England and Wales were attached.[2]

Community psychiatric nurses were becoming a more familiar part

71

of the community nursing service too, so that by 1980 only six districts did not have a service. The spread of community nursing services, however, left a lot to be desired. Often areas where there was clearly a need for such services, because there was either a high proportion of elderly people or insufficient institutional care, were also those lacking adequate community nursing services. Some health authorities employed three times as many district nurses per 1000 population as others while urban areas tended to have fewer attached staff because of lack of accommodation and a larger proportion of single handed general practitioners. The 1974 reorganisation of the NHS, with its emphasis on an integrated approach to health care, obviously made an impact on such inconsistencies.

Differences in training between district nurses and health visitors also threatened to trip up the smooth running of the community nursing services. Since 1948 there had been a statutory obligation to provide health visiting from "qualified women," and their qualifications could be interpreted quite narrowly. In 1962, however, the Council for the Training of Health Visitors was set up, heralding a much broader approach to education and a better understanding of

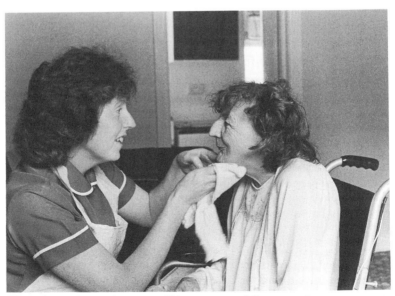

From now on community nurses will have more specialist preparation to meet particular health care needs

the health visitor's role. This body later became the Council for the Education and Training of Health Visitors. Mandatory education for district nurses was not introduced until 1981. Although their training was separate from that of health visitors, it was run by the same body, helping to reduce the differences between the two groups.

Attaching district nurses and health visitors to practices provided a neat solution to some problems and led to better communications— for instance, it inevitably triggered other occupational groups to deal with leadership, the handling of team decision making, and mutual trust and confidence.

Social workers, for instance, who were also becoming attached, wanted to establish their independence, having removed themselves from dominance by doctors in hospitals. Midwives were anxious to maintain their professional freedom, particularly with home deliveries, where the general practitioner could be less experienced than themselves. Health visitors also did not want their autonomy to be undermined and they were concerned that some of their counselling and preventive work did not fit "conveniently" with general practitioners' more curative approach.

So, while the concept of team care was accepted, worries about guarding occupational boundaries and the increasing trend towards specialisation was making it unworkable. Practice nurses were also increasing in numbers.

Where is community nursing now?

Review of services

By 1986 the secretary of state for health in England and Wales commissioned Julia Cumberlege to "study the nursing services provided outside hospital by Health Authorities and to report to the Secretary of State on how resources can be used more effectively, so as to improve the services available to client groups. The input from nurses employed by General Practitioners will be taken into account."[3] The review found a number of weak points and commented particularly on the "separate, traditional ways of working in which health visitors and district nurses appear to be trapped." It took as its focus "the consumer," highlighting three areas of need: people who are dependent want to stay at home; people who prefer to be at home when sick need access 24 hours a day to professional help and support; and people want information about health care and what they can do to prevent ill health and promote good health.

The review challenged the perception of the supremacy of the general practitioner and offered an alternative approach based on giving nurses professional equality and shared responsibility. Overall general practitioners responded negatively, expressing particular concern over the issue of practice nurses and their employment status. The concept of neighbourhood nursing teams and the decentralisation of community nursing services, however, was accepted, and this gathered momentum. By 1988, 36 of 128 district health authorities had developed neighbourhood nursing and 41 were planning to do so. Today community nursing managers are increasingly being involved in the appointment of practice nurses and there are more and more joint initiatives to bring together general practice and health authority staff.

Systems of care

Ninety per cent of contact with patients takes place in the community and it is clear that most people want to remain in their own home and environment. But for the patient community care is a "wheel of misfortune," stuck in a rut of organisational and professional structures (figure). The patient is seen as a recipient of care, and it is very likely that "an endless procession of professionals can enter the patient's home under the guise of quality care."[4]

On the one hand, then, we have the general practitioner, with her or his contractual responsibilities for patients, seeming to be the natural leader of the primary health care team, while on the other is the question of how to make that work when everyone reports back to different organisations.

Where is community nursing going?

Joint working

It is clear that finding the right basis on which to run community health services in general, and nursing services in particular, will be central to the successful implementation of the three government papers *Promoting Better Health*, the government's programme for improving primary health care[5]; *Working for Patients*, the health service in the 1990s[6]; and *Care in the Community: a Consultative Document on Moving Resources for Care in England.*[7] The report of the working group on nursing in the community 1990[8] came at a particularly appropriate time. It emphasises the need for joint working between the district health authority, the family health services

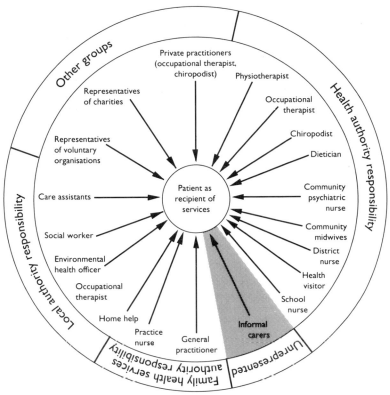

Wheel of misfortune

authority, and the local social services department as purchaser and provider units. For successful joint working, says the report, we will need a shared vision of care; a commitment to joint working and putting patients first; joint assessments of population health needs; joint strategies; effective communications; and a commitment to quality.

Models for community nursing

The report invites discussion at local level around five different models for organising community nursing services with the aim of achieving "the best possible nursing care—within available resources and in the way most suited to the needs of individuals and users and carers."

The "stand alone" community trust or directly managed unit—This

75

model comes closest to achieving good communication and stability among professional staff and would encourage community nursing services to develop marketing and business skills. It could, however, isolate general practice and nursing.

Locality management or neighbourhood nursing—In this model mixed teams of staff are managed in a locality around a geographical patch or a consortium of general practices. This would depend on good networking among team members, who would still report back to different employers—either to the practice or to the health authority. General practitioners could find this confusing, particularly where practice boundaries did not correspond.

Expanded family health services authority—Relationships between family health services authorities and community units with their district purchasing and providing roles would need to be sorted out. In some cases formal links between family health services authorities and community units would be established for the first time. East Sussex family health services authority was in the forefront of the move to build closer working links with community units when it appointed the first nurse adviser in the country in 1988, a practice subsequently followed by others. The obvious outcome of this model is the primary health care authority.

Vertical integration or outreach—This model has a variety of forms including a version that combines acute and community units—for example, mental health units and maternity units might provide inpatient, outpatient, and community services in one provider unit. This model offers "seamless care" for the patient and could shift the emphasis of care to the community, but this could become fragmented. Health promotion and education would need to be estab-

---

Requirements for effective community services

- Joint working and strategies between district health authorities, family health services authorities, and social services
- A commitment to putting patients' and carers' needs first
- Assessments of population health needs
- Preparation and practice so that community nursing, midwifery, and health visiting are responsive to health needs
- Effective communications

lished as the focus could be on those already requiring health care.

The primary health care team — The primary health care team model is centred around a general practice or health centre, with the general practitioner managing all the community services. Its success would depend on skilful team building and setting of clear objectives. The historical divisions among the professional members of the team would have to be broken down and close links forged with secondary care and specialist services.

The report does not champion any one model; rather it leaves it to community nurses and their managers to decide what is right for their own populations.

Current policy and schemes

Current policy on the future of nursing, and particularly community nursing, recognises the need for more flexibility.[9] A new unified discipline of community health care nursing is identified with shared common core preparation for practice and specialist modules to prepare for discrete areas of practice, resulting in greater flexibility of choice for practitioners and employers. In the main the profession has welcomed this development.

The Community Care Act has already had a profound impact on our effort to work along interagency lines. From 1 April 1992 local authorities have had to publish annual community care plans showing what arrangements they are making for community services and community care. In East Sussex the development of care management has a high priority. Six experimental care management pilot schemes have been established, all but one based in general practices and focusing particularly on elderly people and those with physical or sensory disabilities. They are being run initially for one year as a partnership between the primary health care team, East Sussex Family Health Services Carers, and the social services, with the social services as the lead agency. Care management offers the client worthwhile benefits: a single contact point, an assessment of all their health and social care needs, and an overall individual review with regular monitoring. Because the overall amount of questioning and assessing are reduced it is also far less of an ordeal for the client.

Conclusion

Increasingly there is a recognition that although the management and professional issues remain, concentrating first and foremost on what the patient needs is what is helping to break down barriers. Whether a member of staff is attached, detached, or a new recruit is no longer really the critical question. Attitudes, greater clarity about corporate identities, and joining forces to set goals that meet health needs are what count now. It is sharing not protecting, collaboration not isolation, and proaction to health needs not reaction that will make the wheel of misfortune become the wheel of fortune and the patient and carer as involved in setting goals for their own care as are the professionals and managers.

I thank Miss S Mackie-Bailey, proprietor, Gateway Enterprises; Miss D Millward, chief nurse and director of quality assurance, Hastings and Rother NHS Trust; and Mrs P Sinkins, consumer affairs manager, East Sussex family health services for their help.

1 Department of Health and Social Services. *Primary health care: an agenda for discussion.* London: HMSO, 1986.
2 Ottewill R, Wall A. *The growth and development of community health services.* London: Business Education Publishers Ltd, 1990.
3 Department of Health. *Neighbourhood nursing—a focus for care report of the community nursing review October.* London: HMSO, 1986.
4 Griffiths J. *FHSAs: the junior partners? NHS training directorate bulletin.* London: NHS, 1991.
5 Secretaries of State for Social Services, Wales, Northern Ireland, and Scotland. *Promoting better health.* London: HMSO, 1987. (Cmnd 249.)
6 Secretaries of State for Health, Wales, Northern Ireland, and Scotland. *Working for patients.* London: HMSO, 1989. (Cmnd 555.)
7 Department of Health and Social Services. *Case in the community: a consultative document on moving resources for care in England.* London: DHSS, 1981.
8 NHS Management Executive. *Nursing in the community.* London: North West Thames Regional Health Authority, 1990.
9 United Kingdom Central Council for Nursing, Midwifery and Health Visiting. *Report on proposals for the future of community education and practice.* London: UKCC, 1991, 1992.

Caring for the future

MARTIN LAWRENCE

We live in a time of massive change. Primary care is no exception. Having practised in a relatively stable structure since 1948, general practitioners have been affected in the past five years by various government initiatives.[1-8] One thing is certain, the general practitioner is no longer going to be left to practise independently and in isolation. The demand is for accountability—to patients with needs, to a profession dedicated to assuring quality, and to a society which sets targets for effective and efficient care, where possible justified by research. The three areas of accountability are interrelated and the key to satisfying them is partnership.

Patients as partners

It is 40 years since Collings described a practice which had to lock up and bar the door "to stop the patients coming in,"[9] and since the 1966 charter general practice has had the time to evaluate care from a patient orientated standpoint.[10] Byrne and Long described "doctors talking to patients"[11]; Pendleton et al emphasised the need to consider patients' ideas and concerns[12]; but only by 1985 did Tuckett et al acknowledge that the consultation is as much the patient's as the doctor's.[13]

Direct assessment of patients' views and needs has been more difficult to achieve.

Patient participation groups were officially recognised in 1972.[14] They were established with four main objectives: to provide feedback in the planning and evaluation of services; to work with the practice in providing health education for patients (for example, in open meetings or by staffing a patients' library); to act as a safety valve for the transmission and discussion of complaints; and to provide social support (for instance, help with transport for infirm patients). Evaluation of the groups emphasised their enthusiasm but noted that only small proportions of patients participated in the groups.[15]

Community health councils were established in 1975 to provide the patients' viewpoint in planning of the health service. While there was no clear structure for them to use in their early years, the increased role of family health services authorities in planning services has now enabled community health councils to be represented, and many medical audit advisory groups are working with the councils as representatives of patients' views.

The importance of patients' views in audit of care is emphasised by the new contract and encouraged by family health services authorities and medical audit advisory groups. Evaluation is difficult, not least because patients tend to be oversupportive, even in the face of inadequate care,[16] and instruments for eliciting views are currently scarce, usually not well validated, or overcomplicated. Several bodies, both private,[17] charities,[18] and academic bodies,[19] are currently attempting to correct this deficiency.

Assessment of need

Closely allied to the objective of eliciting patients' views is that of assessing need. Patients are able to criticise the care they are receiving,

---

Needs for research and development

- In future it will be necessary to base care on targets and guidelines justified by research evidence

- Adequate tools are required for assessment of patients' needs by the primary health care team

- Research on developing criteria for referral to hospital will enable the development of jointly agreed guidelines between primary and secondary care for the management of common conditions

- There is a need for a mechanism to ensure that the results of research carried out by academic departments are reflected in practice

but it is difficult for them to formulate an unmet need. Any assessment by primary care teams is likely to be partial, owing to lack of expertise in developing instruments for assessment and time and incentive for applying them. To integrate this type of assessment with that of public health physicians would be more informative and realistic.

An example would be the assessment of elderly people. As imposed on practices in the general practitioners' contract this is probably ineffective, but carried out by using the advice of community geriatricians and established tools for assessment[20][21] it could provide a valid and reliable assessment of need.[22]

Partnership in the primary health care team

Total quality management implies that each part of any service is examined by the person concerned with a view to improvement. The primary health care team is ideally placed to undertake such a process.

Consider the management of diabetes. Common failings (with possible solutions) are: inability of patients to make and remember appointments several months ahead (a receptionist can be responsible); deficient review of housebound patients (the district nurse can be involved); feet are not examined (the practice nurse's protocol can be adjusted); glucose control may be poor (the doctor must review the patient's management). At each stage a person from a different discipline knows best how to resolve a problem, what targets are attainable, and what to monitor in order to evaluate success. Practices are learning to work as teams, gaining benefit both in efficiency and morale.

Teamwork in primary care extends far beyond the practice group: district nurses, midwives, community psychiatric nurses, and social workers are developing their own professionalism and cooperating on equal terms. This broad based primary care team, with members exercising their professional capacities, offers a much wider range of care to patients but has a major potential for disharmony unless working procedures are defined. Who, for instance, should advise schools on pupils' smoking—the health visitor, the social worker, the psychiatric nurse, the health education officer, or the general practitioner? Without careful planning areas of community health promotion will be missed as each member of the team leaves it to somebody else: 30 years ago Balint described the same situation in medical care as "the collusion of anonymity."[23]

81

Working together also implies learning together,[24] which leads to mutual respect and full use of special skills. Many practices already arrange "away days"; increasingly, attached staff join in.

Partnership with the family health services authority

Traditionally general practice has operated in an environment with minimal management. This has changed suddenly to a situation where family health services authorities have a very powerful management role. Indeed, all three estates of the law are vested in the authorities—they interpret the rules (legislature), decide whether practitioners have complied (judiciary), and have considerable discretion over payments (executive).

General practitioners' responses tend to be defensive —yet both they and the family health services authorities have the same objectives of better quality care, and family health services authorities and the former family practitioner committees have a long tradition of supportive management of general practice. The uneasy partnership has good reason to flourish.

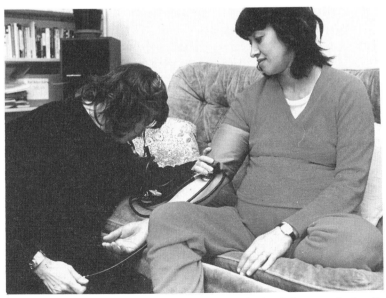

Primary health care workers such as midwives are developing their own professionalism

Arrangements for quality assurance provide an example of a benefit of this partnership. Medical audit advisory groups have an explicit obligation to maintain confidentiality but to provide family health services authorities with the general results of audit.[25] Family health services authorities themselves have a remit to improve quality in their areas. There is increasing cooperation — although the constraints of confidentiality leave the authorities to identify and police unacceptable practice, which they can do both by disciplinary procedures and by using the incentives of discretionary payments.

Partnership and discussion are particularly important if practices are to ensure that their clinical views and particular circumstances are respected. Family health services authorities may issue guidelines, but practices need to agree and adopt precise protocols; and whereas criteria of care can be suggested externally, practices should develop their own standards — as the only external standards that can be imposed are minimum ones. Such practice development with support from the authorities is a key way of improving quality of care. Groups of practices supported by their authorities are working together to influence district health authority purchasing contracts and applying pressure for improving standards. This type of partnership shifts the engine driving quality improvement firmly into primary care.

Partnership with hospitals

The purchaser-provider split can increase the strain between hospital and primary care. General practitioners can shop around for cheaper and better contracts, hospitals can cut costs by reducing prescribing or earlier discharge. There is equally opportunity for cooperation. Fundholding has turned the disincentive to do work in the practice into an incentive, so consultants can reduce their load by developing guidelines jointly with general practitioners, freeing their beds and expertise for more needy cases. Follow up of patients who have had grommets inserted, direct access to hearing aid services, and injection of joints or varicose veins are examples.

Closer cooperation can further increase efficiency. Extensive work is being done on developing criteria for referral, and this will develop into jointly agreed protocols for management of common conditions, which saves patients excessive travel or periods in hospital and doctors the frustration of disagreeing on management.

Emergency work is a grey area between hospital and primary care. Many patients attend the accident and emergency department as their primary care service and some attend for a second opinion. If patients appear to be using the service inappropriately then it is necessary to understand their unmet needs rather than merely to redirect them. For general practitioners to work in accident and emergency departments may be one way of cooperating to solve the problem.[26]

Improved electronic communication will further ease joint management as information will be passed instantly; but problems of confidentiality will have to be faced before a joint record is acceptable between hospitals and primary care.

Partnership in research and teaching

Karl Popper said about Oxford philosophers that they are so busy polishing their spectacles that they never get round to putting them on.[27] But much change in medicine seems to be introduced by people who are unaware that spectacles are available. The new general practitioner contract was introduced after minimal consultation — but since its introduction there has been a rush of academic papers questioning the justification of many of its clinical demands.[28 29]

General practice academic departments are poorly resourced but generate extensive research which should inform current practice. If adequately funded — and the recent provision of tasked money, which is analogous to the service increment for teaching (SIFT) will go some way towards this — they would still need a mechanism to ensure that the results were reflected in practice, politically, through education and across disciplines. At present academics in primary health care are divided, between university departments, regional advisers, the royal colleges, schools of nursing, and so on. Joining these groups into institutes of primary health care, perhaps in one or two universities in the first instance, would develop synergy of effort, ease dissemination of results, and provide a focus for consultation. Such an academic partnership would provide the evidence on which the activities of practical partnerships could be based.

Conclusion

In caring for the population in the future it will be necessary to coordinate the work of professionals and managers, nurses and doctors, employed and self employed, and primary care and secondary care. With such large groups it will be necessary to base care on targets and guidelines justified by research evidence. Patients should benefit from a broadly based primary care team, consulting as appropriate for secondary care services. *The Health of the Nation* encourages health workers to believe that this may take place in an environment which is increasingly health conscious.[8] The reward will be a dynamic approach to health based heavily on primary care.

1 Department of Health and Social Security. *Neighbourhood nursing—a focus for care. Report of the community nursing review*. London: HMSO, 1986. (Cumberledge report.)
2 Secretaries of State for Social Services, Wales, Northern Ireland, and Scotland. *Primary health care: an agenda for discussion*. London: HMSO, 1986.
3 Secretaries of State for Social Services, Wales, Northern Ireland, and Scotland. *Promoting better health. The government's programme for improving primary health care*. London: HMSO, 1987.
4 Griffiths R. *Community care: agenda for action*. London: HMSO, 1988.
5 Secretaries of State for Health, Wales, Northern Ireland, and Scotland. *Working for patients*. London: HMSO, 1990. (Cmnd 555.)
6 Department of Health and Welsh Office. *General practice in the National Health Service. A new contract*. London: HMSO, 1989.
7 NHS Management Executive. *Integrating primary and secondary health care*. London: NHSME, 1991.
8 Secretary of State for Health. *The health of the nation*. London: HMSO, 1991. (Cm 1523.)
9 Collings JS. General practice in England today. *Lancet* 1950;i:555-85.
10 BMA. *Charter for the family doctor service*. London: BMA, 1965.
11 Byrne PS, Long BEL. *Doctors talking to patients*. London: HMSO, 1976.
12 Pendleton D, Schofield T, Tate P, Havelock P. *The consultation, an approach to learning and teaching*. Oxford: Oxford University Press, 1984.
13 Tuckett D, Bolton M, Olson C, Williams A. *Meetings between experts*. London: Tavistock, 1985.
14 Pritchard PMM, ed. *Patient participation groups in general practice*. London: Royal College of General Practitioners, 1981.
15 Richardson A, Bray C. *Promoting health through participation: experience of groups for patient participation in general practice*. London: Policy Studies Institute, 1987.
16 Morrell DC, Evans NE, Morris RW, Rowland MO. The five minute consultation: effect of time constraint on clinical content and patient satisfaction. *BMJ* 1986;292:870-3.
17 *The measurement of patient satisfaction*. London: MOPS Services 1991.
18 *Ask the patient*. London: College of Health, 1991.
19 Baker R. Development of a questionnaire to assess patient satisfaction with consultations in general practice. *J Roy Coll Gen Pract* 1990;40:487-90.
20 Mahoney F, Barthel DW. Functional evaluation: the Bathel index. *Maryland State Medical Journal* 1964;14:61-5.
21 Qureshi KN, Hodkinson HM. Evaluation of a ten question mental test in the institutional elderly. *Age Ageing* 1974;3:152-7.
22 Wilkin D, Hallam L, Doggett M. *Measures of need and outcome in primary health care*. Oxford: Oxford University Press, 1992.
23 Balint N. *The doctor, his patient and the illness*. London: Pitman, 1957.
24 Jones RVH. *Working together—learning together*. London: Royal College of General Practitioners, 1986. (Occasional paper 33.)
25 Department of Health. *Medical audit in the family practitioner services*. London: DoH, 1990. (Health circular HC(FP)(90)8.)
26 Dale J, Green J, Glucksman E, Higgs R. *Providing for primary care: progress in A & E*. London: King's College Hospital, 1991.
27 Magee B. *Modern British philosophy*. London: Secker and Warburg, 1971.
28 Mant D, Fowler GF. Urine analysis for glucose and protein: are the requirements of the new contract sensible? *BMJ* 1990;300:1053-5.
29 Perkins ER. Screening elderly people: a review of the literature in the light of the new general practitioner contract. *Br J Gen Pract* 1991;41:382-5.

Management and administration

SHEILA TEASDALE

Throughout its short history the primary health team has moved through various phases of development. In the sixties the emphasis was on attaching health visitors and district nurses from health authorities. In the seventies and eighties practice nurses came into their own. The nineties will be the decade of the practice manager.[1]

In 1949, 80% of general practitioners worked in singlehanded practices, with no help other than perhaps their wives. In 1989, just before the inception of the general practitioners' contract, 80% of general practitioners worked in group practices,[1] and the current trend seems to be towards bigger practices. In many practices 15-20 years ago the senior receptionist was responsible for the reception area, filing and medical records, and the appointment system, and the doctors took on the management of the other aspects of the practice. Increases in medical knowledge and technology, greater patient expectation, and the demands of successive reorganisations in the NHS have led to an increasing number and variety of staff being employed in general practice. The increased complexity of the organisational structure, along with the more stringent availability requirements of current legislation, means that general practitioners must either manage the staff, resources, and finances of the business in their shrinking spare time or employ someone else to manage the practice with them.

Emergence of the practice manager

During the years leading up to the white papers *Promoting Better*

Health,[2] *Working for Patients,*[3] and *Caring for People,*[4] "practice managers" and "practice administrators" began to appear, but in most practices their true function was administrative. It was recognised that training was needed for these members of staff, and the Association of Health Centre and Practice Administrators (AHCPA) and the Association of Medical Secretaries, Practice Administrators and Receptionists (AMSPAR) both offered training courses covering practice administration and also, though to a lesser extent, management issues.

The real pressure for enhancing the role of the practice manager came from the legislation which followed the white papers. It became imperative to have someone in the practice who could manage the process of implementing the changes required in staffing and working procedures, the financial implications, and so on, and then continue to run the practice effectively, efficiently, and economically. It has to be said that there was some resistance from general practitioners to the change in the practice manager's role—this may have stemmed more from resentment of the imposition of the 1990 contract than from any rational analysis of the situation with which general practice was faced.

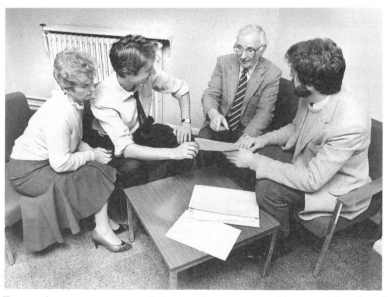

Teamwork among partners and the practice manager enables true delegation of tasks

87

Increasing professionalism

The administrative role within a practice involves implementing and overseeing policy set by the partners, dealing mainly with rules and procedures, and it is essentially a reactive role. In an environment where change is minimal and flexibility and responsiveness to new demands are not required an administrator is a valuable asset, but general practice is in a phase of rapid development which is likely to continue for some time.

There are many definitions of a manager's role: "getting things done through people," "deploying people, resources and money," "planning, organising, monitoring and reviewing," and many more. There is no doubt that any organisation will function more effectively if someone is setting organisational objectives, planning how to achieve them, and monitoring progress towards their achievement, and general practice is no exception. A management role is essentially proactive and requires someone with the ability to respond positively to a changing environment and who can define and agree objectives, analyse problems, establish priorities, negotiate between conflicting demands, devise a strategy, implement the plan, monitor its progress, and review its effectiveness.

A further issue is that managers in small organisations like general practices have a much wider range of responsibilities than managers in large organisations, who usually have only one area to deal with—for example, a personnel manager or a sales manager. In contrast, a practice manager would expect to deal with all of the areas shown in the box.

There has been some development in training available to practice managers to enable them to cope with this expansion of their role: the AHCPA and AMSPAR courses now have a larger management component, and the Open University now offers a distance learning course, "managing health services," which gives practice managers a broader perspective on their role within the rest of the NHS as well as exploring concepts of management in depth.

Some general practitioners still take the view that they do not want to "be managed": this is inevitable, given that one of the reasons why doctors choose to become general practitioners in the first place is that they place a high value on independence and personal autonomy (incidentally, this may also go a long way towards explaining the initial powerful reaction against the imposed changes of the 1990 contract). However, assuming that a practice has employed someone capable of carrying out all the tasks and roles outlined above, what sort of relationship should the partners expect to have with their practice manager?

Relationship with partners

It may be useful to consider the partners as company directors and the practice manager as a managing director: thus the overall aims for the practice are set by the partners, then translated into objectives by the partners and practice manager together, then planned and implemented by the practice manager, and, finally, reviewed by the partners and practice manager together. In this way, the partners are not in danger of feeling that they are losing control of the practice, but at the same time the practice manager is fulfilling a management role, not an administrative one. Working in this way is true delegation: giving a clear task objective with the resources necessary to carry it out and the support to ensure its completion rather than dumping unpopular tasks with no backup. This sort of teamwork is also valuable in that it is visible to the rest of the staff and will thus reinforce the practice manager's authority with them.

The practice manager is a key member of the practice team, and his or her skills are complementary to those of the partners. The practice

---

Management responsibilities of the practice manager

- Patient services
- Quality assurance and audit
- Staffing and motivation
- Internal communication
- Financial management
- Public relations
- Liaison with outside bodies
- Information management
- Legislation
- Systems (design, implementation, and monitoring)
- Premises
- Change

---

manager would not expect to be consulted on clinical matters (unless perhaps they had legal or public relations implications), but would likewise expect the partners not to intrude in management matters where they have been delegated. It is important to ensure that the boundaries of the practice manager's authority are carefully drawn and recorded: in many practices these issues are commonly not made explicit, so the practice manager is unsure of the true extent of his or her remit. This lack of clarity is a common cause of unnecessary friction between the partners and the practice manager. At the same time sufficient opportunities for communication and liaison between the partners and the practice manager must be built into the practice schedule; otherwise the trust so necessary to good working relationships will not develop. It is also important for practice managers to ensure that they are not partial towards any of the partners: the practice manager's job is to ensure the quality of the service offered to the patients and the wellbeing of the practice as a whole.

Staff appraisal

Another factor which complicates the relationships of practice managers within practices is that although not partners, they are responsible for the rest of the staff. This is an isolated, and sometimes rather vulnerable and unsupported position, which can lead to difficulties for practice managers, and hence their practice, if the partners are not aware of problems faced by the practice manager. Management when well done should be "transparent," but it (and the person doing it) thus faces the danger of being taken for granted and overlooked unless something goes wrong.

In many practices one of the tasks of the practice manager is that of staff evaluation, or staff appraisal. This productive technique relies on a positive approach to draw out the skills of the staff and to encourage them to perform better. But who is to appraise the practice managers and motivate them to improve their performance? It is perhaps fortunate that most practice managers are self motivated to a large extent, and the intrinsic challenge of the job itself is enough to keep them working towards their objectives, but staff appraisal is not something which general practitioners can expect to do with no training. The commitment of practice managers who know that they are appreciated and that their talents are recognised will be a dividend which more than offsets the time and cost of learning the skills of appraisal.

Another way of recognising the value of a good practice manager is performance related pay. This can be handled in several different ways: a formula could be agreed by which the practice manager received a set proportion of any increase in profit on top of his or her normal salary, or alternatively a set sum of "bonus" pay could be paid when a particular objective had been achieved (this could be extended to other members of staff also). Some practices have made their practice managers into profit sharing partners after an initial cash investment into the practice by the practice manager, and others have an arrangement where all practice workers, doctors included, divide practice profits equally. Any of these arrangements would secure great commitment from the staff and underline the partners' appreciation of their role in the running of the practice.

Financial management

An area of practice management which has changed and expanded considerably over the past five years or so is financial management. The "market" model and the laws of supply and demand do not sit very comfortably with general practice: the complex structure of remuneration in general practice means that there is often little direct relation between actual hours of doctor-patient contact time and the resulting income, particularly now that government policy places an increasing emphasis on the capitation element. The practice manager must maximise income while at the same time minimising expenditure, as in any other small business, but all the while ensuring that standards of patient care are not compromised.

Financial management is a skill that is often absent in small

---

Necessary skills for a practice manager

• Ability to respond positively to change

• Ability to define objectives, devise strategies, implement plans, and review progress

• Ability to deal with diverse issues

• Communication and liaison skills

• Staff appraisal skills

• Financial management skills

businesses, but the current economic climate forces close attention to be paid to it. The emphasis at the moment is very much on value for money and efficiency. General practice is expected to deliver services of increasingly high quality to patients (or consumers) who are becoming more knowledgeable and articulate, in purpose built premises of a high standard, with specialist staff using up to date medical equipment and computers. At the same time cash limits have been imposed on reimbursement for practice staff and the cost-rent scheme, and the indicative drug amount is a tool designed at the least to increase doctors' awareness of the cost of the drugs they prescribe, though active case finding through health promotion initiatives is likely to lead to increased spending on prescribing. Similarly, bids for resources are now often required by the family health services authority in order to obtain extra funds for developing a practice's services. Preparing a plan of action, collating evidence to support the bid, and preparing the bid itself will usually fall to the lot of the practice manager. Practice managers who do not have experience in financial management need training to enable them to cope with these extra demands.

Implications of fundholding

For practices which are contemplating becoming fundholders in the near future either the existing practice manager will become the fund manager, with extra training if needed, or a fund manager will be appointed while the existing practice manager (if there is one) continues to manage the rest of the practice. The appointment of a fund manager could lead to some conflicts over responsibilities and job boundaries unless these issues are carefully considered beforehand. Fundholding may also have an effect on non-fundholding practices in that patients might transfer to nearby fundholding practices in search of preferential hospital referral unless the service they are offered by the practice is otherwise first class.

The future of the practice manager

Finally, looking briefly towards the future of the practice manager, it is noticeable that the "new breed" of super managers who entered general practice two or three years ago from industry and the services are now beginning to leave general practice. It seems that they saw practice management as a stepping stone to other management positions, and this exposes a fundamental problem for all practice managers and their employers. It is undeniable that there is no real career structure to practice management, other than moving on to a larger practice. This is echoed in the structure of general practice itself: because of the financial repercussions it is very difficult for partners to move once they are established within a practice. This may lead to stagnation and conservatism within a practice unless positive efforts are made to maintain interest. If practices wish to employ managers of high ability who can cope with the many demands and stresses that go with the job they will have to accept that these people, who are likely to be ambitious, will wish to move on after a few years. Alternatively, the practice must find some way of keeping their commitment and interest.

1 Drury M, ed. *The new practice manager*. Oxford: Radcliffe, 1989.
2 Secretaries of State for Social Services, Wales, Northern Ireland, and Scotland. *Promoting better health*. London: HMSO, 1987. (Cmnd 249.)
3 Secretaries of State for Health, Wales, Northern Ireland, and Scotland. *Working for patients*. London: HMSO, 1989. (Cmnd 555.)
4 Secretaries of State for Health, Social Security, Wales, and Scotland. *Caring for people, community care in the next decade and beyond*. London: HMSO, 1989. (Cmnd 849.)

Getting better: education and the primary health care team

R V H JONES

The words "getting better," when applied to any activity, imply that the job to be done is known and that there is agreement as to what is good and bad.

For centuries general practitioners virtually wrote their own job descriptions.[1] It was not until the 1960s that an outline definition was published[2] and the 1980s before attempts were made to define standards.[1] Primary health care teams are an even more recent development. There is still confusion over what constitutes a primary health care team and there are no agreed criteria by which a team's performance can be measured.[3]

In most practices, however, there is a recognised group of people —general practitioners, district nurses, practice nurses, a manager, health visitors, and clerical and secretarial staff—who normally work together from the same building to service the health needs of the same registered population. At a time when more practices are analysing what they are doing and looking at what the results are and what they would like them to be it is appropriate to consider the educational needs of these teams and how education may improve their performance.

Educational needs of individuals

It is usually assumed that the professional education of nurses, health visitors, midwives, therapists, social workers, and general practitioners has equipped them for work within primary care. This

94

may well not be so. Moreover, before their appointment to a practice, few practice managers, receptionists, and secretaries had until recently trained for their jobs in a medical context. In addition to filling basic educational gaps continuing education in the form of updating knowledge or of learning new techniques and skills is essential for everyone working in primary health care.

For staff employed by a practice the responsibility for recognising and meeting their educational needs rests squarely with the general practitioner. This applies to all staff but is particularly important for practice nurses, most of whose daily work has not been covered during their professional training. For professional staff attached to practices but employed by health authorities responsibility rests with the authority. Health authorities differ in the extent to which they acknowledge this responsibility, and difficulties concerning funding and protected educational time for attached staff can arise as they participate more in audit and educational activities in the practice.

Educational needs of the team

The members of the primary health care team, with their diverse skills, roles, and tasks, have in common that they work within the same organisation and that collaboration and cooperation is a major aspect of their work.

In the past general practice was carried out by an individual doctor

---

Requirements for adult education

Adult education should:

- Be relevant (directly related to daily work)
- Be learner centred (meet learners' needs)
- Be problem based
- Be interactive
- Build on learners' experience
- Challenge learners to commit themselves to a decision
- Provide a logical approach
- Provide feedback
- Lead to further study

working in isolation. The importance of understanding the principles of management and their relevance to maintaining high standards of performance and motivation[4] have only slowly been appreciated by general practitioners, as small practices have turned into medium sized businesses.[5][6] Most general practitioners learnt nothing about management during their medical education, and neither did their staff. Although practice management is now an integral part of vocational training, there is a need for continuing education.

Another consequence of the increasing size and complexity of general practice has been that the need for good teamwork has become more evident. The recent shift of emphasis from hospital to community care for people with long term disability and incurable disease, together with increasing realisation of the complex implications for service of an aging population, have sharply focused attention on the current deficiencies in teamwork within primary health care teams.

Meeting educational needs

Skills

There is no one method for meeting educational needs: needs are different, people are different; some may appreciate one educational method, others heartily dislike it. However, updating basic knowledge and skills through courses with lectures and discussion or with supervised practice of skills are appropriate and effective. Most health professionals feel comfortable with this familiar, non-threatening method. Courses along these lines are regularly advertised in professional journals and organised in postgraduate centres.

Management

Advertisements for management courses also appear in professional journals. As consensus agreement is an important component of successful change in management attendance by both a practice manager and a general practitioner partner is encouraged for most management courses.

Teamwork

The most difficult educational need to meet has proved to be that of improving teamwork. Improved teamwork requires a new awareness of colleagues' skills, roles, and expectations and changes in attitude and behaviour. Traditional "teacher centred" educational methods have been shown to be ineffective in changing behaviour among general practitioners.[7] In searching for an effective method[8] the emphasis has shifted to "learner centred" education,[9][10] in which the teacher's role is largely that of a facilitator. Surveys of mature students[11] and research into motivation of adults in education[12] have shown that adult education should fill the requirements listed in the box.

Methods and models for improving teamwork

As a means of improving teamwork learning together—multi-professional education—should in theory be more effective than learning about each other at a distance. Take up of multiprofessional workshops if advertised as such, however, has often proved disappointing (British Postgraduate Medical Federation, personal communication). More recently several educational initiatives entailing members of different health professions cooperating in a joint task have proved more successful. The three examples of educational methods described below had different objectives, but one common outcome was improved teamwork.

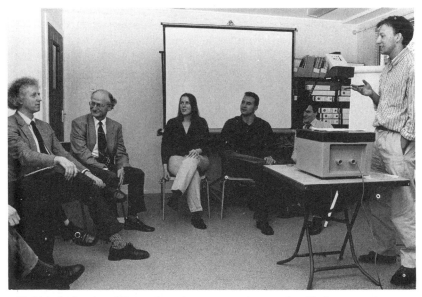

Multiprofessional workshops adopt a learner centred approach, with the tutor acting as a facilitator rather than a lecturer

(1) Facilitators in primary care

In the Oxford region nurse facilitators were employed in a research project concerned with preventing coronary heart disease and stroke.[13][14] Their function was to advise and work with practices in a screening programme. Although the main objective of the project was to improve preventive care, it was found that coordinated planning and cooperation within the practices had increased.

(2) Multiprofessional workshops

For some years the Lisa Sainsbury Foundation has been running one day workshops, which have been largely uniprofessional. There was a demand for certain subjects to be considered in greater depth, and since 1990 the foundation has organised some residential workshops on terminal care at home. To broaden the perspective within a workshop each interested practice should nominate both a nurse and a doctor to attend. The format of the courses is interactive, with the tutor acting as a facilitator rather than a lecturer. Feedback has been positive and the courses are fully booked.

(3) Residential practice workshops

From 1987 Yorkshire Regional Health Authority, the regional adviser, Yorkshire Heartbeat, and the Health Education Authority have organised a series of residential workshops for general practices. The main aim was to reduce the incidence of coronary heart disease by encouraging health promotion in general practice. Other aims included encouraging understanding among professionals and team-work. The programme has been fully described[15] and evaluated.[16]

Each practice nominated its own team of four to six members to attend, which might typically include a practice nurse, general practitioner, social worker, district nurse, health visitor, and practice manager. The main objective was that by the end of the workshop each practice would have produced an agreed plan of action, which they would implement. During the course most time was to be spent in practice discussion interspersed with short contributions providing information about, for example, local resources or the need for the plan to include evaluation and ways of doing this.

The programme has gradually developed. The main objective that each attending practice should produce a plan remains, but the content of the plan has broadened to include topics chosen by the practice. Attendants during courses have shown increased understanding and tolerance within practice groups.[17] The response from participating practices has been enthusiastic. Evaluation has confirmed that in most practices the plans have been introduced successfully and that improved teamwork persists. These and similar workshops are now widely available.

Common features

Despite different origins in different settings and different objectives these three initiatives share common features—namely, that as educational exercises they are all learner centred, interactive, build on the learner's experience, and are relevant in that they relate to real problems or challenges in daily life. They have each included more than one profession or discipline, and as a result of each better cooperation, more coordinated planning, and improved teamwork have occurred.

Back to the practice

Of the three examples described, one involved a facilitator; in the other two members of the practices attended workshops outside the practice, thus gaining protected time. But similar opportunities can arise or be organised within the practice itself. In a recent article Essex and Bate describe an audit within their practice.[18] They conclude that the method they developed enabled a receptionist to audit aspects of the practice cost effectively and that there was great scope for enlarging the receptionist's role. It is interesting to analyse the process which led to this conclusion from an educational viewpoint.

The first reported action was a decision to audit accompanied by the setting of goals by the medical partners. The receptionist and partners met regularly to identify difficulties. When insufficient information was available the receptionist conferred with the relevant doctor, health visitor, or nurse. The receptionist participated in redesigning the forms for collecting data. In effect within an audit exercise a multiprofessional interactive educational exercise took place in which a practice team were working together to solve a problem relevant to their daily work, the problem being quality control.

Education is generally accepted as an essential component of audit. Perhaps in general practice there is a mirror image: audit of a practice activity which concerns several professions provides an excellent and often unrecognised opportunity for multiprofessional education, better understanding, and joint planning.

Key points

• All general practice staff have a need for continuing education

• The general practitioner is responsible for meeting the educational needs of staff employed by the practice

• The health authority is responsible for meeting the educational needs of the staff it employs

• Multiprofessional workshops are effective in improving collaboration within primary health care teams

• Audit of practice activity by several team members may be the best way of improving teamwork

---

Maybe it is time the focus shifted from going away to learn to learning at home. The potential is there. Clearly the need will arise for comparison with others,[19] but as a first step in "getting better" it is worth consideration. Resources and guidelines are available. Many local medical committees and faculties of the Royal College of General Practitioners can provide help and guidance. Each family health services authority has its medical audit advisory group, which is able to provide advice and perhaps some initial funding. Perhaps it is time that medical audit advisory groups themselves became multiprofessional.

Conclusion

While some members of primary health care teams have basic educational needs all have the need for continuing education. This requires time and money. Health authorities differ in their willingness to accept responsibility for the staff they employ. Unfortunately many general practitioners are still unwilling to provide enough time and money for educating their staff, which is a strong disincentive for their motivation and effectiveness.

The major challenge, however, is to improve collaboration and cooperation within primary health care teams and between these teams and other health and social service professionals working in the community. Multiprofessional workshops with practice teams have been shown to be effective, but audit of a practice activity that requires the participation of several team members is a potent method of improving understanding and cohesion—members work together and learn together.

1 Royal College of General Practitioners. *What sort of doctor: assessing quality of care in general practice.* London: Royal College of General Practitioners, 1985. (Report from general practice 23.)
2 Royal College of General Practitioners. *The future general practitioner learning and teaching.* London: BMA, 1972.
3 Jones RVH. Teamwork in primary care: how much do we know about it? *Journal of Interprofessional Care* 1992;6:25-9.
4 Drucker PF. *The practice of management.* London: Heinemann, 1955.
5 Pritchard PMM, Low KB, Whalen M. *Management in general practice.* Oxford: Oxford University Press, 1984. (General practice series No 8.)
6 Jones RVH, Bolden KJ, Pereira Gray DJ, Hall MS. *Running a practice.* 3rd ed. London: Croom Helm, 1985.
7 Horder J, Bosanquet N, Stocking B. Ways of influencing the behaviour of general practitioners. *J R Coll Gen Pract* 1986;36:517-21.
8 Jones RVH. *Working together—learning together.* London: Royal College of General Practitioners, 1986. (Occasional paper No 33.)
9 Knowles MS. *The modern practice of adult education: from pedagogy to androgogy.* Cambridge: Adult Education Company, 1980.
10 Brookfield SD. *Understanding and facilitating adult learning.* San Francisco: Jossey-Bass, 1987.
11 Woodley A, Wagner L, Slowey M, Hamilton M, Fulton O. *Choosing to learn: adults in education.* Milton Keynes: Open University Press, 1987.
12 Rogers J. *Adults learning.* 2nd ed. Milton Keynes: Open University Press, 1977.
13 Fullard E, Fowler G, Gray M. Promoting prevention in primary care: a controlled trial of low technology, low cost approach. *BMJ* 1988;294: 1080-2.
14 Fowler G. Coronary heart disease prevention: a general practice challenge. *J R Coll Gen Pract* 1988;38:391-2.
15 Lambert DMD. *Team workshops for health promotion in primary health care organised by the Health Education Authority for the prevention of coronary heart disease.* London: Health Education Authority, 1988.
16 Spratley J. *Team workshops for prevention and health promotion in primary care organized by the Health Education Authority: evaluation report.* London: Health Education Authority, 1989.
17 Jones RVH. Working together: a description of residential multi-professional workshops. *Postgraduate Education for General Practice* 1990;3:154-9.
18 Essex B, Bate J. Audit in general practice by a receptionist: a feasibility study. *BMJ* 1991;302:573-6.
19 Pringle M. Newark information sharing project: lessons for medical audit advisory groups. *Health Trends* 1991;23:15-8.

Beyond the boundaries: relationship between general practice and complementary medicine

PATRICK C PIETRONI

Traditional medical partnerships were designed to operate in a stable unchanging environment. It is clear that the next five years will be neither stable nor unchanging within primary health and community care. General practitioners for the first time are operating within a managed health service, and the autonomy they once had to determine their administrative routines is rapidly disappearing.

These changes will inevitably challenge the organisational structures currently found in general practice. Inevitably, nurses, social workers, counsellors, midwives, health visitors, and dieticians will demand a place within an integrated health care team, and general practice will have to adapt. At the same time the increasing popularity of some of the complementary therapies will continue and we will have to address the question as to their relevance to the delivery of care within the community.

Relationships between general practitioners and complementary practitioners

Definitions

One of the problems faced in exploring the relations between general practitioners and complementary practitioners is that there is no clear definition of words such as "alternative," "complementary," "holistic," "natural," and "fringe," which are often used to describe vastly dissimilar activities. Much confusion arises from the belief that holistic medicine and alternative medicine are the same thing. There are as many general practitioners who apply the principles of a holistic approach to their patients as there are acupuncturists who do not. The term "alternative" or "complementary" medicine is used as a catch all definition for anything not taught at a Western medical school. It is thus a definition by exclusion and as helpful a term as "foreign." An Englishman setting out to comment on "foreigners" would be as accurate in his description of foreigners as most doctors are in their understanding of alternative therapies, and the Englishman's commentaries on foreigners would tell us more about the prejudices of being English than the characteristics of non-English people. The classification that I find most helpful divides the vast subject of complementary therapies into four distinct areas[1]:

- Complete systems
- Diagnostic methods
- Therapeutic modalities
- Self care approaches.

Some of the methods that fall into these categories require four years of full time training akin to undergraduate medical school, while others can be learnt and applied after a few weekend seminars. It is inappropriate and does reasoned debate an injustice to lump all these categories together under one definition and respond with a prejudiced or enthusiastic stance.

It is outside the scope of this article to examine the burgeoning field of complementary medicine, but it is clear the general practitioner will require some guidance from an authoritative and unprejudiced

---

Examples of treatments in four areas of complementary therapy

Complete systems
Homoeopathy, osteopathy, herbal medicine, acupuncture

Diagnostic methods
Iridology, kineseology, hair analysis, aura diagnosis

Therapeutic modalities
Massage, shiatsu, reflexology

Self care approaches
Meditation, yoga, relaxation, dietetics

---

source before deciding which treatments to consider including in their expanded primary health care service. Research at Marylebone Health Centre has begun to provide some guidance.[2-4]

The growth of complementary medicine

A survey in the United Kingdom in 1982 identified a total of 30 000 complementary practitioners of one sort or another.[5] Subsequent developments have suggested a growth of 10% a year, which would make the present figure nearer 50 000. The consumer magazine *Which?*, in its survey of almost 2000 readers, found that one in seven had visited a complementary therapist in the past year.[6] A survey undertaken by the Market and Opinion Research Institute (MORI) in 1989 showed that 74% of the sample surveyed (1826 adults) would have liked to see some form of complementary medicine introduced into the health service.[7] The interest among general practitioners has increased in the past 10 years. Reilly found a positive attitude towards complementary medicine in 86 of 100 general practitioner trainees in 1982,[8] and Wharton and Lewith, in their survey of 200 general practitioners in the Avon district, found that 38% had received some additional training in one form of complementary therapy.[9]

Clinical outcome and research papers in several areas of complementary therapy now find a place in orthodox medical journals, and it is no longer possible to maintain the traditional medical stance that referring patients to complementary therapists is unethical. The pressure for including some form of complementary therapy within the health service will continue to increase as a result of the King's Fund report on osteopathy.[10] In a recent open letter the junior health minister supports the view that general practitioners can employ complementary therapists in their practices as long as they retain clinical responsibility.

Power, conflict, and collaboration

This history of "outsider" or "alternative" medicine is as long as history itself. It could be said that for a while general practice was viewed as alternative medicine or as an unacceptable alternative to medicine. Many of us were told that we were selling ourselves short, we had fallen off the ladder, if we embarked on a career in general practice. Lord Moran's comments on the establishment of the Royal College of General Practitioners in the 1950s still rankles with senior colleagues. "Over my dead body," he said. General practice, of all disciplines, should be sensitive to the views of colleagues in complementary medicine who experience the same arrogance and ignorance from doctors. But the antipathy goes much further back and the language is much richer, as the following description from the seventeenth century shows.

> But our Empirics and imposters, as they are too ignorant either to teach or to practise Physic . . . and too insolent, and too arrogant to learn of the Masters of that Faculty, or to be reduced into order: so are they most dangerous and pernicious unto the Weale public. . . . These Crocodiles, disguised with the vizard of feigned knowledge and masking under the specious titles of Physicians and Doctors, not attained in Schools, but imposed by the common people, do with the Absolonicall Salutations steal away the affections of the inconstant multitude, from the Learned Professors of that Faculty, with their loablike Imbracings, stab to the heart their poor and silly patients, ere they be aware of once suspect such uncouth Treachery.[11]

More recently, studies undertaken at Marylebone Health Centre have shown a less fraught but equally difficult pattern of relations

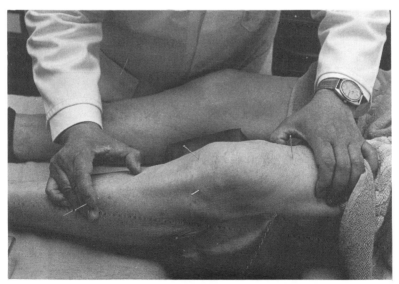

It is no longer considered unethical to refer patients to complementary practitioners

between general practitioners and complementary practitioners. Issues identified in these studies included the following[12] [13]:

• The variety of clinical models informing the different practitioners, which led to different assumptions about outcome

• The nature of the referral process and the power issues implied by the general practitioner acting as the only gatekeeper

• Organisational conflicts that arise out of the appropriate allocation of resources (rooms, funds, secretarial help, etc)

• Empowerment of patients and the subsequent disempowerment of practitioners.

No one group can hope to resolve these problems, and more research is required before recommendations about the integration of complementary medicine into general practice are made.

Options for changes

The following are some possible options for the integration of complementary medicine into general practice.

Traditional

Ancillary staff funding by family health services authorities—Complementary practitioners can now be employed like any other ancillary staff if general practitioners can persuade the family health services authority to provide the reimbursement. They operate within the health centre, in a similar manner to physiotherapists or counsellors—that is, patients are referred by general practitioners, who retain clinical responsibility. All complementary practitioners employed at Marylebone Health Centre (practitioners in massage, osteopathy, acupuncture, herbal medicine, and homoeopathy) operate under this model. Levels of pay are determined and set by the practice to reflect experience and status—for example, massage practitioners are on the same scale as a clinical nurse specialist and osteopaths are on a clinical assistant grade. The family health services authority reimburses 60%-70% of their pay and the rest is supported through health promotion reimbursement (this will change following recent legislation).

Privately funded—Complementary practitioners are referred patients privately, in a similar manner to other specialist services. Some practices have provided free space within the practice for private work in exchange for two to three NHS patient referrals a week. Other groups have shared premises and have cross referrals from both groups.

Research studies to explore the use of complementary therapies in general practice are now more easily funded and it is possible to receive both regional and district funding for such activities (the work at Marylebone Health Centre began in this way).

Local fundraising activities—The need to develop services through charity and voluntary contributions begs many questions, yet it can prove to be the only way in which services can be supported. Several groups have employed complementary practitioners in this way.

Direct funding—Some district health authorities and family health services authorities have employed osteopaths, massage practitioners, and counsellors directly themselves and then seconded them to those practices that are in a position to make use of them. Fundholding practices are clearly able to do this themselves.

Practice placements—Marylebone offers a six months' massage training course during which time the candidates have to work for 40 hours in a general practice. These practice placements are "free" and offer both the student and the practice an opportunity to explore and develop experience in their particular therapy. Links with other training establishments are currently in progress to expand this scheme.

Primary health care referral centre—Many practices wishing to cooperate with complementary practitioners are unable to because of lack of space. One health authority is exploring the possibility of providing a referral centre for five or six practices from which com-

---

Key points

• There is a need to define precisely the various terms used when referring to complementary medicine

• Many areas of complementary medicine are now accepted by patients, some general practitioners, orthodox medical journals, and politicians

• Possible ways of integrating complementary medicine and general practice need to be explored

• Integration could be traditional, with the general practitioner retaining the role of sole gatekeeper, or could be part of a move towards a multiprofessional practice

---

plementary therapy, counselling, and other additional services can be provided.

Experimental

All the previous models maintain the traditional relationship between the general practitioner and the complementary practitioner—that is, the general practitioner retains clinical responsibility and acts as gatekeeper in the referral process.

We are currently experimenting with a model where the patient is given the option to choose whether he or she sees the general practitioner or goes directly to a complementary practitioner. A further experiment is that of the dissolution of the general practitioner partnership as the core to the structure of health care teams. The proposed model of a multiprofessional practice would involve some of the following possibilities:

- All clinicians and senior administrative staff would share ownership of premises

- Decision making would be delegated to a practice management group to include:

    one general practitioner selected by all the general practitioners
    one administrative member of staff (practice manager)
    one other clinician selected by the non-general practitioner clinical staff

- All clinical and administrative staff would be on salaried contracts, to reflect experience, status, qualifications, etc, and hours of work

- Profits would be shared equally among all staff and based on length of service and performance related indicators

- Medical accountability and liability would be a corporate and not individual concern

- Patients would be registered with the "practice" and not with the individual general practitioner.

This model will not appeal to many general practitioners struggling to maintain their autonomy and status, but the logic of all the recent NHS reforms points in this direction. My view is that although our roots may lie in medical schools and our current identity is that of general practice, our future lies as members and, at times, leaders of an expanded primary health and community care team which, among others, must include selected complementary practitioners.

1 Pietroni PC. Alternative medicine. *Journal of the Royal Society of Arts* 1988:791-801.
2 McLean J, Pietroni PC. Self-care—who does best? *Soc Sci Med* 1990;**30**:591-6.
3 Peters D, Davies P, Pietroni PC. Osteopathy in general practice: a year's audit. *J R Coll Gen Pract* (in press).
4 Deeser A, Davies P, Chase D, Pietroni PC. Traditional Chinese medicine in general practice: an audit of one year's referrals. *J R Coll Gen Pract* (in press).
5 Fulder S, Monro R. *The status of complementary medicine in the United Kingdom.* London: Threshold Foundation, 1981.
6 Magic or medicine? *Which?* August 1981.
7 Mori Poll. *Times* 13 Nov 1989.
8 Reilly D. Young doctors' view on alternative medicine. *BMJ* 1983;**287**:337-9.
9 Wharton RW, Lewith G. Complementary medicine and the general practitioner. *BMJ* 1986;**292**:1498-500.
10 King's Fund. *Report on osteopathy.* London: King's Fund, 1991.
11 Beier LMcC. *Sufferers and healers—the experience of illness in seventeenth-century England.* London: Routledge and Kegan Paul, 1987:38.
12 Reason P, Chase HD, Desser A, Melhuish C, Morrison S, Peters D, *et al.* Towards a clinical framework for collaboration between general and complementary practitioners: discussion paper. *Journal of the Royal Society of Medicine* 1992;**85**:161-3.
13 Reason P. Power and conflict in multidisciplinary collaboration. *Journal of the Research Council for Complementary Medicine* 1991;**5**:144-50.

The developing primary care partnership

MIKE PRINGLE

It is clear that if a clean start could be made, primary health care teams would probably look substantially different from the ones we encounter today. The historical development of primary care has resulted from three concurrent pressures—political, organisational, and clinical.

Development of primary care

The existence of primary care teams can be largely attributed to the 1966 charter, which also limited the range of skills available within the team. The rules for reimbursing 70 per cent of staff costs defined eligible job descriptions; if that list had included physiotherapists, social workers, or counsellors the nature of primary care itself over the past 25 years would have been radically altered. The recent relaxations have given practices much more discretion but have also introduced the possibility of a lower reimbursement.

The second pressure has been organisational. The moves towards group practices, practice reports, audit, and computerisation have all emphasised the need for administration and management. The increasing sophistication of practice information systems for managing both clinical care and the resources of the practice has reached its apotheosis in fundholding. Practices joining this scheme require a level of internal organisation that would have seemed unachievable and unbelievable a decade ago.

Perversely the increasing management role in primary care has resulted in less involvement in management by some doctors. The arrival of practice managers with high level skills has freed general practitioners from administration and often from direct management responsibility. The increase in clerical staff has given the practitioners support with paperwork that their colleagues of 1966 could only envy.

The third major pressure derives from clinical evolution. In recent years there has been an accelerating transition of medical care into general practice. Child immunisation, developmental assessment, and family planning have been shared with agencies in district health authorities, but the 1990 contract has often led to their transfer to primary health care teams. The national surveillance of the "healthy" population through well person clinics, visits to the over 75s, and new services such as foreign travel clinics has augmented the workload and responsibility of primary care.

Through the 1980s there has been a shift in the care of patients with chronic disease from secondary care into general practice. The closure of many psychiatric hospitals, with the transfer of their longstay patients into the community; the move to offer routine management of many chronic illnesses—for example, hypertension, asthma, myxoedema, diabetes, and epilepsy —in general practice, which has removed most of these patients from hospital follow up; and increasing open access to pathology and radiology services and treatments such as physiotherapy and minor surgery, has reduced the requirement for hospital referrals.

These three historical trends have clearly created the head of steam that has driven the primary health care team forward for nearly

---

Key points

- The primary health care team as we know it has developed largely in response to political, organisational, and clinical pressures
- Education is required for team members deficient in necessary skills
- The personal responsibility of each member within the team framework must be identified and accepted
- Patients should encounter the teams, not unconnected coworkers
- Every member of the practice should participate in quality assurance
- The result of effective teamwork should be, primarily, an increased quality of care

30 years. In the process many serious structural and process problems have been created, which we ignore at our peril.

Current problems facing primary health care teams

What is a team? A team is more than a list of coworkers in a practice report, although that may vary widely. If a team is to mean anything it must embody a method of working, a process not a structure.

In all too many practices the team rarely meets. Care is transferred between team members with the minimum of consultation and tasks are delegated without proper communication and education. All too often protocols for major diseases are written by doctors without team discussion, but implemented by practice nurses without training.

Qualifications and skills

Some team members have been recruited with inadequate qualifications. Some practice nurses are ill equipped for their job, and many dispensers are barely trained receptionists. Deficiencies in skills result in reduced self confidence, and then a loss of respect within the team. So a first strategy must include improved standards in staff appointments allied to education for those in post.

Once all team members are secure in their skills they need to be valued. Only if their opinion is sought, and reacted to, and they are then involved in implementing subsequent changes, will practice team members feel as if they belong to a real team.

Real teamwork

Increasingly practices will examine whether clinical care is really given by a team or individuals. Even antenatal clinics—a paradigm for interdisciplinary working—are often only a method of duplicating effort, with genuine dual consultations being rare. Many "health promotion" protocols for monitoring diseases entail doctors and nurses seeing patients separately. If the team approach is to be a reality the patients must encounter teams, not just unconnected coworkers, each with clearly defined areas of interest.

Doctors and nurses often choose to work in primary care because they value their autonomy. They seek and prize a personal responsibility direct to the patient. The ethos of working in a team conflicts directly with this desire for autonomy, and this tension needs to be acknowledged and discussed. Only when all team members can identify their personal responsibility within the team framework, and are comfortable with that allocation, will "the team" be given more than lip service.

This in turn requires the leadership role to be shared. The general practitioners, traditionally the owners of the practice in every sense of "ownership," understandably often see themselves as the employers with the ultimate control. They may dispense some power, but only conditional on their ability to retrieve it when necessary. The perceived and tangible hierarchy in general practice perpetuates the status of nurses, practice managers, and attached staff as coworkers rather than team members.

Educational needs

Another problem concerns the educational needs and experience of team members. The doctors have their needs recognised and encouraged by the postgraduate education allowance, but practice nurses and managers are dependent on the goodwill of the practice and the whims of the family health services authorities for their educational needs being met. When education occurs it is common for team members to undertake it separately.

Audit

The last major problem concerns quality. Medical audit is slowly establishing itself, but it needs to be widened to include all the clinical, managerial, and administrative members of the team. It may be satisfactory to start by auditing the medical content of a diabetic clinic, but the nursing input also needs auditing, as does the appointment availability, the timing of the clinic, the information given to patients and their satisfaction, and, of course, the outcome. Everybody, including the receptionists, needs to be involved in such quality assurance.

Auditing will have a positive feedback on performance only if the responsibility for the work and the results are shared among those concerned. If tasks are delegated without information, training, and support the team member cannot then be held accountable for the result.

Future possibilities

Financial rewards

Many of these problems will be addressed as primary care evolves. Fundholding practices in particular are undergoing a culture change to one that values every patient contact, and will increasingly raise the status of all team members. All practices will eventually confront the need to offer more than psychological rewards to all key team members. Performance related pay is increasingly being discussed, but few practices have found a satisfactory formula. The definition of "performance" is problematic, as is the nature of the reward.

One solution which seems to be gaining credibility is to offer key members of staff—practice managers and nurses, for example—a partnership share. Although this share would not be equal to that of a medical partner, it would allow all senior team members to share in increases in practice profitability by having a mutual stake in increasing income and controlling expenditure.

Nurse prescribing

As nurse prescribing moves up the agenda, wise practices will realise the implications for indicative drug amounts and fundholding budgets. The more the nurse feels ownership of the practice's finances the more likely is nurse prescribing to relate harmoniously to that of the doctors.

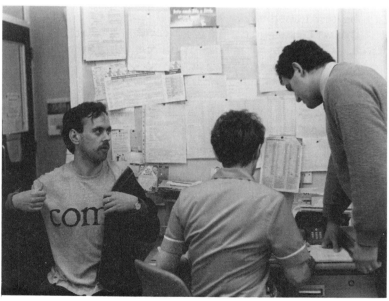

Real teamwork entails patients encountering teams and not, for example, seeing doctors and nurses separately

Community nurses

It seems probable that community nurses will become more integrated, not less, with the primary health care teams, perhaps as practice employees, or, more likely, as community unit employees subcontracted to the practice. Only practices that have a good system for integrating and valuing all their staff will succeed in welcoming the currently attached staff into full team membership.

Changes in attitude

By redefining the definition of a "partner in the practice" the structural problems in motivating senior members of the team may be overcome. But the behavioural problems will remain. Doctors will increasingly have to accept the primacy of others in areas where their skills are traditionally less developed, in particular in nursing and management. The problems of integrating some team members up into the centre of the practice will be mirrored by the problem of integrating the doctors down into the centre.

A good place to start is the identification of common tasks and the requirements to meet or improve the performance of those tasks. The requirements may be educational or managerial, clinical or organisational. By working together towards common goals team members can learn to value each other.

For most practices this will not require outside experts—facilitators, management consultants, or gurus—but internal re-evaluation and discussion. If an event such as changes in staff is used to trigger this process then the practice needs to be primed to react positively. At present the most common precipitant is fundholding, but this need not be the case.

The end result should not simply be better work relationships or even greater financial efficiency, although both of these are laudable. If the primary health care team is to achieve anything it must increase the quality of health care. The evidence for its success must therefore rest on the services offered and their standards. This is the holy grail to be unearthed by the attitudinal, cultural, change ahead.

Conclusions

Given a clean start, nobody would create the structure and process of the current primary health care team. If we can espouse a coherent vision of the future for the team, such as has been put forward in this series of articles, then methods for evolving towards it can be found.

115

The key element in this vision of the future is that all team members must be valued as skilled professionals in their own right. That implies responsibilities—on them to gain and retain skills, and on the practice to motivate them—but it does not imply wholesale structural change. New organisational techniques will be needed and the notion of "partnership" redefined, but if the primary health care team of tomorrow is to work it must be characterised by quality caring— quality caring for patients and quality caring for each other. That is easy to conceptualise but, like all cultural changes, difficult to make happen.

Index

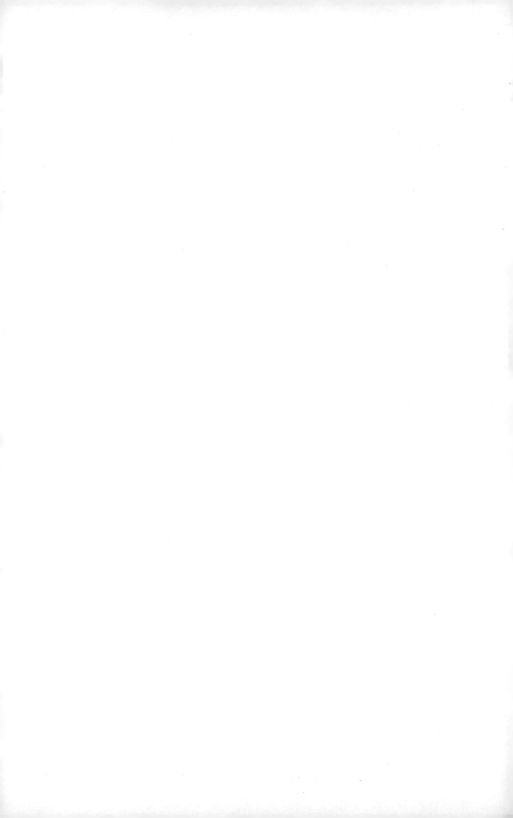